HELP, HOSPIT/
AND
THE HANDICAP!

HELP, HOSPITALS AND THE HANDICAPPED

Aspects of the Practice of Clinical Psychology

DAVID F CLARK

ABERDEEN UNIVERSITY PRESS

First published 1984
Aberdeen University Press
A member of the Pergamon Group

© David F Clark   1984

British Library Cataloguing in Publication Data

Clark, David F
　Help, hospitals and the handicapped
　1. Mentally handicapped – Care and
　treatment
　I. Title
　362.3'8   HV3004

ISBN 0–08–030377–3
ISBN 0–08–030402–8 Pbk

Printed in Great Britain
The University Press
Aberdeen

CONTENTS

Preface		vii
Acknowledgements		ix
I	INTRODUCTION	1
II	THE CLINICAL PSYCHOLOGIST'S CONTRIBUTION	8
III	SENSORY MOTOR TRAINING	19
IV	INSTITUTIONS AND THE PSYCHOLOGIST	42
V	ASPECTS OF BODY IMAGE	70
VI	PSYCHOTHERAPY: AN EXERCISE IN ECLECTICISM	90
	Bibliography	115

PREFACE

This book is for anyone who is prepared to utilise all available resources in a flexible way for the benefit of the mentally handicapped, who will remain open-minded about new policies and who will be prepared to found his or her ideas and practices on a basis of active discussion and firm knowledge.

There are many graduate and under-graduate psychologists, psychiatrists and other professionals, as well as members of the general public with special interest in handicap, who need to have appropriate background information—a source book—for their interest and activity in helping and understanding the mentally handicapped.

The review nature of sections of this book, interspersed as it is with new material deriving from the author's own current work, will make it of particular value to post-graduate students of clinical psychology and psychiatry who are preparing not only for examinations but, more importantly, for daily practice involving some of the issues and skills discussed.

Two other groups were in the writer's mind when the book was prepared. Nurses in psychiatry, mental handicap and community care, and also social work staff are increasingly being urged to play a larger and more active part in caring for the handicapped in the community. Hostel and Adult Training Centre supervisory staff and care personnel now seem likely to bear as much of the burden of fighting off the effects of institutionalisation in their own smaller community units as has been borne by psychologists, psychiatrists and nurses in hospitals for the mentally handicapped during the past twenty years or more. It is hoped that people in these categories will find in some parts of this book a starting point for ideas and skills in the management of clients, staff and care units generally, also for setting up rational and congenial client training programmes, and for effective counselling when necessary.

In recent years the most popular expressions in the literature on mental handicap have been 'community care' and 'normalisation'. There can be no denying the rights of the handicapped to both of these but there should be more thoughtful consideration as to whether merely by establishing these rights we ensure optimal living conditions for the handicapped. The best exercise of these rights must necessarily be guided and facilitated by a range of skills and supports, and these may be provided in a variety of ways. The best hospitals offer less institutionalisation, more enrichment and more highly skilled and often specialised care than do many small community homes and hostels. The guardian or the foster parent may still need the help of the nurse, the teacher or the psychologist, and there is no fundamental reason why hospitals should not be as much part of the community as are churches, schools or day centres.

As for 'normalisation', one may ask whether this should mean the same for a moderately handicapped Down's Syndrome man from a remote Shetland croft; for a behaviourally disturbed 18-year-old girl from the more depressed area of an industrial city, or for an orphaned middle-aged spastic with no speech from a family of deep sea fishermen? There are dangers in being too much beguiled by catch-words.

D F Clark

ACKNOWLEDGEMENTS

The author is greatly indebted to Dr Thomas S Ball and his publishers, C E Merrill Publishing Company, Columbus, Ohio for permission to quote a section of his book *Itard, Seguin & Kephart: Sensory Education, a Learning Interpretation* and to Frederick Busch and Scotsman Publications Ltd for permission to quote the whole of his poem 'What the Body Says'.

The author would like to express his warm gratitude to his secretary, Mrs Frances Raymond who has shown great tolerance, forbearance and skill in typing the several drafts necessary before the final production of the separate chapters. He would also like to acknowledge the friendly collaboration and stimulus of his professional colleagues in all disciplines at Ladysbridge Hospital, Banff, which has made his work there so worthwhile and contributed in a variety of ways to some of the content of this book.

CHAPTER I

INTRODUCTION

It is often hard to predict, particularly in the behavioural sciences, how some sort of balance may emerge in one's professional work between a steady, and sometimes rather wearing, commitment to clinical work with patients and specific problems of practice demanding detailed research solutions. Indeed this balance can usually be effectively assessed only with hindsight and may be determined by several chance factors—colleagues, setting, opportunity and so on. Some issues, however, fall between these activities, research and practice, in the sense that both conduce to the occasional review of salient ideas or procedures. Often, the opportunity for such an explicit revaluation of tacitly held ideas occurs in the context of national and other conferences or in discussion with post-graduate clinical psychology students, psychiatric and nursing colleagues. The writer is indebted to many of these for both their support and their criticism. With the exception of the one on body image, which is more of a research paper, the five essays which make up the body of the book emerged from conference and occasional lecture presentations of that kind. They are intended to encourage an interest in the richness, complexity and variety of work which is available in the field of mental handicap for a number of disciplines but especially clinical psychology, psychiatry and nursing and to reflect something of the width as well as the depth of interest which clinical psychologists are currently finding in what has traditionally been thought to be a rather unrewarding field of clinical and research endeavour. In spite of the trend in care of the mentally handicapped to the community rather than the hospital there remains a need for the input of informed, highly skilled and committed professionalism from the disciplines mentioned, and from others not referred to in particular, to *both* clinical settings. The goals and principles of care and treatment will remain the same.

It is a luxury of any research or academic appointment that the holder may focus his efforts on some specific problem or field of work and research. The practising clinician, on the other hand, seldom enjoys such single-minded dedication to any particular topic or style of work and has, like the skipper of a sailing ship in a gale, to yield to immediate pressures and to handle crises with the equipment and knowledge available at the moment. Experience may enable him to extemporise or experiment within limits but the immediate demand characteristics of the job determine the parameters of such efforts. For that

2   HELP, HOSPITALS AND THE HANDICAPPED

reason, the five following chapters take the form of papers and lectures, longer than would be appropriate for publication as articles in learned journals, but each representing some aspect of the thinking and research to emerge from a variety of features of one practitioner's daily work with the mentally handicapped. They make no claim to be inclusive. Some important studies of psychological work with the handicapped, many, like behaviour modification, for example, the stock and trade of the writer, are omitted, either because they have been published elsewhere by the same author or better and more fully by other authors.

There is also a 'general' quality about these papers, an attempt to deal with broader issues, which often can be lost in the style, compression and commitment to data which technical journal articles favour. This is perhaps more apparent in some chapters than in others. For example, the chapter on body image is heavily data-based but is aimed nevertheless at pointing up broader similarities in the way in which the handicapped as well as we ourselves evaluate our own physical characteristics. By contrast, the chapter on institutions and the psychologist is entirely discursive but draws elements from sociological and social psychology literature which are important to those who work in institutions whether these be hospitals, hostels or day care centres.

To some extent also, the topics dealt with in these essays are the product of the context and style of operation adopted by the author. Ladysbridge Hospital, Banff, in which he has worked for the past 18 years, unlike the large urban institutions which were his former stamping grounds, has gone through several evolutionary phases in the course of each of which certain determinants of the content of the subsequent chapters emerged. The hospital started its life in 1866 as a general 'asylum for lunatics', a 288 bedded Victorian edifice geared entirely to containment and seclusion from the community. It was staffed by nurses and 'warders' long before it sported a medical superintendent and nearly 100 years before it greeted its first clinical psychologist. However, considerable reorganisation of mental health services within the then North-East Regional Hospital Board in Scotland during the 1950s and 1960s saw the old Ladysbridge Hospital with its special wards for chronically sick and tuberculous psychiatric patients disappear in favour of a whole new campus of buildings planned for the long term care of the mentally handicapped.

Attitudes within the Health Board at that time were also very favourable to a psychological, as distinct from a psychiatric, input to the care and treatment of the mentally handicapped. The Chairman of the Board and the then Medical Superintendent, in appointing in 1966 a Consultant Clinical Psychologist rather than a Consultant Psychiatrist anticipated by nearly a decade and a half the Peters Report and in so doing flung a stone into the pond of clinical psychology, the ripples from which later lapped the shore of the established view in a generally satisfactory way. It is true that there had been centres of outstanding and sometimes pioneering work in clinical psychology in mental handicap before this. One thinks in particular of the important work of the Clarkes and their associates at the Manor Hospital, Epsom, and of Gunzburg at Monyhull Hospital near Birmingham. History will confirm the debt which the mentally handicapped owe to these innovators in rehabilitation theory and practice, since developed by Mittler both when he was a clinical psychologist in the National Health Service and later with his team as Director of the Hester Adrian research centre in Manchester. This writer has certainly no hesitation in acknowledging his considerable personal debt to all of these. The important difference in the development in Grampian, however, was that in this instance a Consultant Psychiatrist was being replaced by a Consultant Psychologist rather than the latter supplementing the former, as was the case in these other institutions.

The report, 'A Better Life', a report on services for the mentally handicapped in Scotland (1979) eventually caught up with the viewpoint expressed by the North-East Regional Hospital Board 13 years earlier when in paragraph 7.62 it felt able to say, 'The contribution of clinical psychologists in the field of mental handicap is well established: in intellectual assessment and in the investigation of perceptual and speech anomalies, in devising, in initiating and monitoring schemes of behaviour modification and in work in association with educational psychologists. There is a clear need for additional personnel in this field, and as with other para-medical professions we believe that the scarcity of clinical psychologists in this field is partially due to the relative neglect of this work in the training of clinical psychologists'.

That Report and its earlier English equivalent 'Better Services for the Mentally Handicapped' (1971) contributed heavily to a more forward looking and enlightened approach to the care of the mentally handicapped. While both Reports stressed the importance of a wide range of facilities for this special population they agreed that the long term institutions—and hospitals in particular—had an important part to play in their care and treatment. It is perhaps worthwhile quoting again from the Peters Report (para 7.25) the defining characteristics and functions of a hospital in the context of a comprehensive service for the mentally handicapped. These functions are:

(1) To provide specialised diagnostic and/or assessment procedures.
(2) To provide a range of therapeutic techniques, including medical, nursing, psychological, physiotherapy, speech therapy, occupational therapy and social work facilities, in a coordinated therapeutic programme, individually designed to enhance and develop the physical, emotional, social and intellectual capacity of each patient, with a view to the development of their full potential, and to enable them to achieve a positive and independent life, in so far as their handicap permits.
(3) To provide long term care in a protected environment for those incapable of leading an independent life, e.g. persons with severe

physical handicap and/or severe emotional/behaviour disorders who require constant nursing care and supervision.

(4) To provide secure accommodation for patients with mental handicap and associated anti-social behaviour of such a nature as to require the protection of the community.

(5) To provide short term institutional care to meet specific individual or family needs, such as intensive re-training and rehabilitation, or holiday admission to give respite to parents. This last function should diminish in importance as alternative resources become available.

(6) To ensure facilities for education (including further education), training, and recreation for all patients.

The view encapsulated there was broadly the conception of the role of the hospital for the mentally handicapped held by the author on his appointment in 1966. Institutions, especially when they are a century old, however, develop an ethos and climate of their own and a number of elements in the situation therefore conspired to limit the extent and speed of any change toward the goal of putting that conception into practice. First, the hospital was one which was staffed by people who had a long tradition of nursing in their families but many of whom were trained in general and psychiatric nursing with a strong bias toward custodial care rather than in nursing for the mentally handicapped. Cleanliness and order, routine and the hierarchy were therefore main concerns and the notion of the institution as a home where people with a condition were cared for rather than as a series of wards where people with diseases were treated was hard to inculcate. Second, the notion that by being the largest employer in the district, the hospital should be a relatively unchanging institution with certain fixed characteristics was firmly endorsed in the minds of those working for it. This too inhibited change and the re-deployment of staff in particular. Thirdly, the hospital staff at all levels were unused to having a clinical psychologist—and certainly one at this level of seniority—around the place. Previously, a relatively junior clinical psychologist from the Department in Aberdeen braved five hours in a bus to work for a couple of hours once a week on what inevitably became only routine assessments. It took a number of years before an attic room was replaced by a purpose built Psychology Department and more before another purpose built building for occupational, industrial therapy and patient training could be constructed. Meanwhile, the psychologist, after completing a first assessment of all the patients, was progressively able to introduce patient activity programmes, behaviour modification, group discussions and therapy sessions, ward rounds and staff meetings as well as to accumulate appropriate staff assistance. It was this process, deliberately undertaken then, and still far from perfect in its achievement or aim, which encouraged the author in his view that the clinical psychologist in such a setting will only be effective if the 'professional', 'executive' and 'social engineering' roles outlined in Chapter 4 are fulfilled.

Similarly, the need to establish patient activity programmes and a system of sensory motor training for the many patients heretofore neglected or limited to ward life, drew attention to what the literature had to say on the topic from its early beginnings with the Wild Boy of Aveyron to the nearly domesticated animals of the laboratory and the relatively tame psychologists of the 1970s. Chapter 3 derives from that need and demonstrates that theoretical problems remain. These are largely concerned with what mediates change in sensory and motor behaviour and in what terms that is to be measured. There is less doubt among practitioners about the intrinsic value of such programmes of stimulation, communication and activity to the patient's own sense of involvement with others and of personal worth.

One of the major conflicts which engage psychologists in their planning of patient training programmes generally lies in the choice, often in a situation where both staff and money resources are in short supply, between setting up detailed personal programmes for patients with special needs and organising a general kind of tick-over programme which will occupy all patients in a less specific way. Often the attempt to compromise in this leads to anomalies in the level of patient care in particular instances and to difficult decisions about which patients key resources should be directed toward. The cost effectiveness of particular programmes of care and training or treatment is an area which has, so far, received all too little systematic research.

Such research needs, perhaps, to be at several levels. In the first instance, there needs to be costing of what is the best, both in terms of economy and effectiveness, kind of staff, number of staff and physical equipment to achieve for the mentally handicapped an enjoyable and stimulating life. Such an accounting exercise can be realistic, however, only if there is a reliable method for estimating the gains experienced by the recipient as well as by the donor of the training, bearing in mind that the criteria that such recipients may adopt in estimating improvement may differ greatly from those adopted by their mentors. Another related issue to this which deserves more thoughtful reappraisal is concerned with how far one is justified in 'prescribing', especially for adult or elderly handicapped persons, every or even most of the details of their activity or scope for activity each day. Of course one supposes that the very old will almost automatically lapse from 'training programmes' just as one makes similar assumptions about babies and the very young, but how often do we ask the mentally handicapped what sort of care they want; and how often are we not trapped into specifying, prescribing and ordering on the medical model of treatment òf a disease rather than that of caring for a person? The Mother-knows-best syndrome was irksome enough to us, even if valid, as children and it normally tends to lapse by the time we reach our teens. Thirdly, there requires to be some philosophical scrutiny of how far it is reasonable, as well as charitable, to go on disbursing public funds in favour of the mentally handicapped group with its limited productivity rather than to spend in favour of the unemployed, the chronically sick or the intellectually gifted. Naturally, those of us who are intimately concerned with caring for the mentally handicapped have few doubts about where our sympathies lie. And in a rich and advanced civilization there should be no question but that all its ailing or deprived members should get the help that is necessary for them. In times of economic stringency, however, some of these issues stand out more starkly and certain lines, even if tenuous ones, may have to be drawn. Writers in the technical press have tended to shy away from such issues but even these must be subject to rational analysis and adequately researched solutions.

Many issues of the above kind recurred in individual and group therapy sessions with the mentally handicapped which had been run by the author. Perhaps the very concreteness of the thinking of that group kept the Reality Principle very much to the fore and led inexorably to the eclecticism in psychotherapy advocated in Chapter 6. It is in such situations, especially in group therapy and at their own activity groups and social clubs, that the essential human qualities of even the severely handicapped shine through. Given that transience of mood and shortness of immediate memory-span limit expression of their feelings and views, there is always in them a residual need for, and giving of, affection, a sympathy for those even worse off than they, and a sharpness of perception of the shallow and insincere, deriving from a variety of perceptual sources, which is impressive. Bodies, however stunted and deformed; movements, spastic or coordinated; and sensations blunted by paralysis or other pathology are nevertheless evaluated consistently by their owners. The emotional evaluative aspect of body image maintains its integrity even in the face of enormous disrupting forces. The handicapped lives in our world as we do in his. How he perceives himself in it is, in this respect, reassuringly similar to our own self-perceptions, as Chapter 5 shows. What the author has not explored and what others may care to research is the developmental nature of body image as it is progressively formed through childhood and adolescence. Up till now the main research by the writer and others has preoccupied itself with adults where skeletal growth is complete. Just as we know how body image has to adapt to traumata like amputation and paralysis so also there is much to be learned about the growth of our identity in body terms which remains obscure. As the writer has pointed out elsewhere (Clark, 1975) our bodies allow us to express our sense of personal identity in so many ways as well as allowing us to develop it, that it is surprising that it has not been the subject of more detailed research. As we struggle to develop more and more complex man/machine interfaces of an electro-mechanical and electronic sort and as more and more prosthetic devices and organ replacements occur we should perhaps be looking carefully at our conception of body image and fitting these heroic endeavours rather more exactly to what is already known.

If these speculations should seem to have veered away somewhat from the field of mental handicap, it is simply to illustrate how many and varied are the ramifications of working as a clinical psychologist with that group. As in a general psychiatric setting, the clinical psychologist has to live with the conflict between working as a scientist in his research and analysis of ideas and as an artist in his care and curing techniques. A few can settle unequivocally to one or the other task. Most, however, who are not full-time researchers or academics, settle for compromise and switch hectically, and sometimes anxiously, between these two roles. Perhaps the ideal to strive for is a situation where skilled and professional manpower is sufficiently available to staff units or departments with groups of each—a cadre of applied scientists who care and cure and a cadre of purely research oriented scientists who live and work with the former, closely and intimately enough to stimulate, inform and enthuse each other with the variety and adventure of their work. Meanwhile the relatively few clinical psychologists in the field of mental handicap struggle away in both roles, their mobility severely limited by having a foot in each camp. At least the clumsy steps they have taken so far have been of some direct value to their handicapped friends, and have created a body of knowledge and good practice which, by being reinforced or criticised, can only enhance our claim to being civilised.

CHAPTER II

THE CLINICAL PSYCHOLOGIST'S CONTRIBUTION

Any attempt to write briefly on the historical background of clinical psychology in mental subnormality often seems to carry the implication, hinted at if not specific, that one has oneself experienced an epoch of change in which the elements have been lived through rather than read about. Unfortunately, this is all too true in that the writer is reminded that some 26 years have passed since he published his first paper in mental subnormality (Clark, 1958), even though he was not working specifically in that field at the time. There is a constant need, therefore, to shrug off the somewhat dyspeptic, 'I've seen it all before', outlook on what has gone by and at the same time avoid a surfeit of overenthusiasm for one's special or idiosyncratic interests.

It is proposed here to select a number of general trends which seem to reflect the diverse activities of a wide range of clinical and academic psychologists who have looked at the problems of the retardate on both sides of the Atlantic. Inevitably, a number of seminal papers will be disregarded and some famous names omitted. For that, the writer must crave the reader's and those authors' pardon. Nor is it proposed to dwell on the not inconsiderable contribution of a number of eminent psychiatrists in mental deficiency, many of whose contributions have been informed, humane and often psychological.

As a first statement, it will be all too evident that the contemporary Zeitgeist in psychology is such that no longer is a preoccupation with psychometrics and mental measurement crucial to an *understanding* as distinct from definition and categorisation within mental deficiency. The trend is now more toward the prediction and control of individual behaviour and occasionally of groups, through the planned manipulation of institutional and/or environmental conditions. This is clearly reflected in the day to day activity of most clinical psychologists in mental deficiency settings, in that the Wechsler, the Stanford Binet, the Progressive Matrices, the Minnesota Pre-School Scales and so forth are now less frequently wielded than PAC, Adaptive Behaviour scales and individually styled behaviour analysis sheets for individual patients. Clearly this is not to denigrate entirely the value of formal intelligence testing. The usefulness of such tests with the handicapped has been debated by, among others, Baumeister (1965), McAndrew & Edgerton (1964) and Ross & Boroskin (1972). However, for purposes of primary classification standardised intelligence tests do have a predictive function and, of course, correlate well with one another even at the low end of the distribution. There may well be difficulties of standardisation at the lowest end of the curve but a more significant defect is that scores on intelligence tests can be seen only as a partial description of behavioural functioning. The formal test is fundamentally a predictive, administrative device rather than a guide for treatment (Baumeister, 1965). Moreover, it is the common experience of clinical psychologists that a large number of handicapped people, in long stay institutions particularly, will not be practically testable in this sense and many psychologists like Landesman–Dwyer (1974) would feel that the variability of response in such populations is something which may be of more significance than absolute level, particularly at the lower ability levels. One is inclined to agree with Schmitt & Erickson (1973) that perhaps the most useful feature of standardised assessment of intelligence lies in the early definition and identification of individuals who may benefit from intensive training whether this be (preferably) in early childhood or subsequently.

Berkson and Landesman-Dwyer (1977) have indicated that, building on the philosophy of the Vineland Social Maturity Scale and similar scales, there is now a preoccupation with assessing adaptive behaviour which has to some extent supplanted a lot of the enthusiasm for traditional intelligence testing. They quote a number of references for the development of this fairly elaborate technology and outline some of the difficulties involved. Their review suggests that, on the whole, certain dimensions seem to be agreed on as representing important functional areas where psychologists can become more effective measurers. These are in ambulation, self-feeding and table manners, dressing and grooming, toileting skills, activity level, stereotyped and self-destructive behaviour, anti-social behaviour and social communication. They point out at the same time that the main function of scales developed to measure these variables is to identify areas for training and levels of success of such training rather than a continuation of the predictive and administrative function for which intelligence tests were developed. Such an approach follows, of course, a much more idiographic than nomothetic model.

Perhaps the greatest influence in transforming the clinical psychologist in handicap from a measurer to a treater and trainer partly derives, on the one hand, from an awareness of the sterility of measurement as such, and on the other from a detailed critical scrutiny of what we have become used to call 'the medical model'. The Clarkes (1977) have recently indicated that the latter may well be very appropriate for the reduction of the incidence of handicap in the very severely retarded of so-called pathological type, although they are rightly less sanguine about the effectiveness of such techniques as amniocentesis, genetic counselling and an understanding of the genetics of inborn disorders of metabolism, as being able, of themselves, to reduce the occurrence of mental retardation by 50% before the end of the century in the way that the USA's President's Committee on Mental Retardation predicted in 1972. More importantly, there has been an increasing concern with the effects of modified environment on behavioural development especially with the retarded. A series of studies both with animals and humans in the past 20 years have demonstrated that early experiences can retard or promote an individual's development in a very significant way even when nature has determined the wider or narrower limits within which this may occur. Bricker (1970) succinctly reflects this view when he expresses his belief 'in the importance of the nervous system,' (coupled with) 'a conviction that a host of events can do damage to its functioning. However, only the failure of a perfectly valid, perfectly reliable, perfectly efficient programme of training will convince me that the identification of the deficit is sufficient reason to stop trying to educate the child'.

The new enthusiasm, therefore, for education and behaviour modification reflected a fundamental shift in the strategy of psychologists looking at handicap. The methods they have used have been borrowed from the principles of learning theory that were first expressed by Hilgard, Hull, Spence and others in the early 1950s. At that time we knew psychologists were somewhat in awe of terms like 'stimulus/response', 'reinforcement schedule', 'generalisation' and so forth. They were thought to be the concern of the psychology department library and the more abstruse textbooks that dogged our final examination years. However, as Berkson & Landesman–Dwyer (1977) indicate, by the middle 1970s such terms no longer had anti-humanistic and mechanistic connotations but represented more the main conceptual tools for changing the behaviour of the retarded. As a consequence, there have been spectacular achievements based on the application of such technology. Berkson & Landesman-Dwyer (1977) have reviewed this in some detail and workers who are involved in this field will know better than the writer the most appropriate references to reflect the change in general strategy. It is adequately reflected in journals and texts by Gardner (1972), by Thomson & Grabowski (1972), by Schaefer & Martin (1969), and more recently by Yule & Carr (1980).

The kind of self-help skills that have been taught using learning theory approaches include standing without support, walking instead of crawling, avoiding life endangering activities such as chronic regurgitation and a whole variety of self-feeding skills, including table manners as well as manipulation of table tools. Patients have been taught to dress themselves, to brush their teeth, to use sanitary towels and obviously to cope with the details of toilet training. Other important areas include the reduction of anti-social behaviour, self-injurious behaviour, stereotyped rocking and picking, screaming, pica, hyperactivity, head banging and so forth. Many of these programmes have been initially experimented on by small groups of clinical psychologists interested in the particular behaviour in question but carried forward by applied psychologists in institutions on both sides of the Atlantic and revalidated on many occasions. The aboriginals, so to speak, of this work must necessarily be Pavlov, Skinner, Hull, Guthrie, Tolman, Solomon & Wynne and so forth. They are the theoreticians and original experimenters whose path we applied scientists have subsequently trodden and eventually beaten into something more like a royal road to behaviour modification for the handicapped.

There are, however, several problems encountered in such programmes. These mostly relate to such issues as individual variability and acquisition rates (which is yet another aspect of the increased variability found in so many characteristics of the subnormal in general), the finding of suitable reinforcers, the programming of task sequences, failure to generalise beyond the training situation and, perhaps more damning, a lack of follow-up after initial training, together with the very significant ethical and moral problems arising in the application of aversion techniques. There must be enough research material in these topics alone to occupy most clinical psychologists in the field.

As such a strategic change occurred in the activities of clinical psychologists in handicap, so also did the style of experimentation change to include not only a scrutiny of populations and groups defined in terms of IQ and chronological or mental age, but toward the single case experimental design (Hersen & Barlow, 1976; Kazdin, 1975). In this the wheel turns almost full cycle to the earliest days of psychologists' interest in handicap, when Itard was so diligently tackling the deficiencies of Victor, the Wild Boy of Aveyron.

Those who are interested in the mainsprings of sensory education of the handicapped could do worse than look again at Ball's (1971) book on Itard, Seguin and Kephart. Ball analyzes Itard's efforts in terms essentially of instrumental learning and the orientation reaction. At the same time he tries to relate how Itard & Seguin went about their work in relation to the more recent work of Kephart (1968). While acknowledging that there was 'an amazing serendipidy' in Itard's work, Ball takes the view that the serendipity arises from the fact that, from the conclusion of his initial effort at stimulating the senses to the beginning of reading instruction, Itard pursued a programme of sensory training which, according to Kephart's theory, represented a seriously inappropriate teaching strategy. Judged from Kephart's standpoint it was severely inappropriate for two basic reasons: (1) it ignored the sensory motor component as a foundation for the learning process, and (2) it focussed on a type of discrimination training that emphasised a narrow specificity and seemingly impaired the development of perceptual organisation and conceptual generalisation. However, it is Ball's view that it is precisely because of these misdirected perceptual training efforts that we are able to see the subtle and far-reaching implications of perceptual training today.

Kephart's work itself represents a cognitive approach to the interpretation of the mediation of learning difficulties in which he describes a series of increasingly efficient strategies for processing information from the environment. These stages must be learned sequentially, and, according to him, if learning at an earlier level is incomplete, learning at higher levels must inevitably suffer. In this way his theory resembles that of Piaget (1952) but he is also indebted to Hebb (1949) in that Kephart is more prepared to establish a neuro-psychological model through which he accounts for the disruption which occurs in the learning process of the disabled learner. While his theoretic rationale for treatment strategies comes largely from Hebb and also perhaps from Strauss and Lehtinen (1947) many of his practical remediation procedures reflect the influence of Maria Montessori (1964) who in turn was strongly influenced by Seguin. Kephart draws heavily upon hypothetical constructs, i.e. inferences about actual events that go on inside the organism between stimulus and response. Another factor that differentiates him from the Skinnerians and places him in Piaget's camp is his emphasis on the motor component of intellectual development. According to Kephart, at the earliest stages the child's information processing strategy is largely motor in nature. If his motor patterns are not properly developed he is not likely to be able meaningfully to contact and apprehend the world about him. In later stages, the motor component becomes subservient to the child's evolving perceptual and conceptual capacities but Kephart would go so far as to suggest that, in the first instance, intellectual deficiency is tantamount to a disrupted and undeveloped motor system. Following these views, contemporary psychologists have been much concerned to develop programmes of sensory motor training as a necessary adjunct to a more direct cognitive/perceptual training programme. Readers of Ball's book (1971) will find an interesting parallel drawn between the work of Kephart and that of Zaporozhets (1965) in Russia. The whole business of developing sensory experience, of cross modal matching and of the linking of motor activity to cognitive apprehension has been jointly supported by the work of Zaporozhets, of Luria and by the animal studies of Held & Hein (1963, 1967), Held & Bauer (1967) and cognate studies of babies by White & Held (1967). It was that early work which laid the foundations for a series of studies on the most appropriate content of sensory motor training programmes such as those by Ruth Webb (1969), Maloney, Ball & Edgar (1970), Ball & Edgar (1967) and those critically examined by Morrison & Pothier (1972). (See Chapter 3 of this volume).

The fact that even severely and profoundly handicapped people can have their behaviour modified appropriately and their level of skill and self-help increased by such programmes encouraged a number of psychologists, in this country particularly, such as Tizard, O'Connor, Hermelin, Claridge and the Clarkes to look more carefully at the abilities and trainability of dull people and the more moderately handicapped. The results of this work of the early 1950s are well known in that formal programmes of sensory discrimination, literacy and the development of industrial skills are now well developed and can be attributed directly to the early reports of these psychologists. In a sense, of course, a great deal of preliminary work at the laboratory and experimental level had been undertaken by such people as Ellis (1963) and his associates who were probably among the first to study operant conditioning extensively in the more severely retarded (Barnett, Ellis & Pryer, 1960; Ellis, Barnett & Pryer, 1960) to say nothing of his fundamental work on stimulus trace deficit

(Ellis, 1963). Similarly, eminent researchers like House (1973), Zeaman, House & Orlando (1958) and House & Zeaman (1958) contributed to an understanding of discrimination learning in the retarded which is of lasting importance. These workers adumbrated the persisting difficulties of establishing generalisation from a learned response after training in a particular response. Berkson & Landesman-Dwyer (1977) in their recent review therefore consider the literature on transfer of training to be particularly signficant, so that studies on learning sets, transfer, imitation and verbal mediation in the handicapped are of some importance. They quote a series of references for those concerned but conclude, among other things, that fading is a powerful technique for training new skills and effecting transfer (Bricker et al 1969; Dorry & Zeaman, 1973) and that teaching a person to imitate the teacher's response and coupling the imitation with verbal instructions tends to increase the behaviour repertoire fairly rapidly. Yet again, however, imitation may be limited to the trained response class and is sometimes again not subject to generalisation. They also go on to indicate the importance of language in intellectual activity and social interaction (Barton, 1973). A few psychologists like Hollis & Carrier (1975) are working on non-verbal communication but there is lots of room for further work with individuals who have no overt language and who might learn non-vocal communication. There is scope for fruitful collaboration between speech therapists, psychologists and teachers of the deaf in elaborating the use of Makaton and other signing systems with the handicapped. The writer and his clinical colleagues are currently pursuing this.

A further mainstream group of psychologists should perhaps receive honourable mention. In some ways we can group these together as the Normalisers and those who have looked carefully at institutions and institutionalisation. Among the former are those who have committed themselves heavily to a scrutiny of the nature of the lives of the handicapped both in naturalistic settings and in large and small institutions and who have attempted to reassert the place in the community of the moderately subnormal and to enrich the lives of the more severely subnormal wherever they are. The names of Gunzburg (1968), Wolfensberger (1972) and Nirje (1970) immediately spring to mind as psychologists who have been concerned to humanise in an enlightened and scientific way both the activity programmes, the living conditions, the learning skills and the personal experience of the handicapped at all levels. Those who wish to re-read some of the seminal papers in this connection should look at the book edited by Gunzburg (1973) where Gunzburg's own preface will give a different kind of historical overview from this and where several chapters will illustrate very well the progressively changing philosophy which has underwritten a great deal of the practical work of clinical psychologists subsequently. As he says, 'If the institution is to provide experience to further the aims of habilitation, it follows that its climate, environment, the rhythm of living and the occupation and leisure activities, should be as near life as possible to be preparatory to the stage of comparative independent life in the open community and to counteract the faulty and inadequate experience of the past.' This is a much more careful statement following Nirje's (1969) original pronouncement on normalisation than that found, for example, in the recent Jay Committee Report.

Any statement which sees normalisation as 'providing experience to further the aims of rehabilitation' is allowing more flexibility in the definition of the term than perhaps its originators anticipated. It is, however, important for the rehabilitator, be he psychologist or not, to recognise the inherent paradox of normalising when the subjects of that process are by definition subnormal or abnormal in respects which may in some cases not be amenable to substantial change. Moreover, in preparation for life in the open community it must be remembered that the survival skills, values and even the measures of success for many of the mentally handicapped are going to show considerable variation between those characteristic of a middle class suburban environment, a deprived and crowded inner city slum and a Shetland croft. So what does normalisation really mean for the handicapped person who is to be prepared for discharge into one of these? The issue is simpler for those who remain in the hospital, hostel or group home.

It would be impossible also to go past this point without recognising too the dominant influence of Allan & Anne Clarke (1974), in Great Britain, as psychologists who started as clinicians in hospital and finished as academics writing in much more general terms but who have never forgotten their concern for the individual handicapped person. Their experimental work and writing, especially on development stages and deprivation, has been illumined by academic stringency, theoretical rigour and care about details, as well as by a humanitarian concern for their subject. In many ways they can be said to have orchestrated, through their books and papers, the efforts of many more service-oriented clinical psychologists the length and breadth of the country and abroad.

While the theory of normalisation derived great impetus from people like Gunzburg and Wolfensberger there can be no doubt that the sociologists Goffman and Pauline Morris have played their part also, and stimulated the work of other psychologists such as King, Raynes & Tizard (1971), Zigler & Balla (1977), and McCormick, Balla & Zigler (1975). Not the least valuable piece of work that King, Raynes & Tizard (1971) carried out was their extensive and sensitive cross-institutional study of residential care practices in institutions for the handicapped in England.

In the course of this they developed their resident management practices inventory which has become a useful measure of the social/psychological characteristics of institutions. This instrument was conceptualised as tapping institution-oriented care practices at one extreme and resident-oriented practices at the other. As many will know, the items in the inventory could be grouped along four dimensions of rigidity of routine, block treatment, depersonalisation, and social distance. The first was concerned with the inflexibility of management practices so that at one extreme neither individual differences among residents nor unique circumstances would be taken into account by staff in their interaction with patients. So far as 'block treatment' was concerned, the regimentation before, during and after specific activities such as games or mealtimes, was obvious, and 'depersonalisation' was a measure of the presence or absence of opportunities for residents to have personal possessions, privacy or situations allowing self-expression and individual initiative. 'Social distance' was concerned with the limitation of interaction between staff and residents to formal and specific activities and the use of physically separate areas of congregation between the patients and those who cared for them.

Now that it is a contemporary issue to discern what is the best type of care for the handicapped, such investigations can go far to pointing up good and bad practices. It must be recognised by many psychologists that small units, whether run by social work or health service agencies, may be every bit as institutional as large units and that what seems to be important is type rather than size of institution in determining the style of care practices. When Zigler & Balla (1977) replicated this type of study in the States, they found that while in large living units size and level of retardation were found to be predictive of institution-oriented rather than resident-oriented care practices, they also found that cost per resident per day, the number of aide staff per resident or number of professional staff per resident did not predict care practices. This was an important finding since apparently simply increasing expenditure or personnel will not of itself necessarily guarantee better styles of care for the retarded, rather it is how these staff are utilised in the settings. This finding perhaps bears an important message to most of us. The flexibility, warmth and resident-oriented attitudes of staff are much more critical determinants of style of care.

The final influence worthy of report at this time is perhaps itself a combination of many of these already animadverted on. The Clarkes in the 1950s indicated that proper programming of learning and proper incentives and knowledge of results could transform the skills of moderately and some severely retarded people. In the following decade behaviour modification, as has been already indicated, developed as a formalised system and was involved in care programmes. More recently, however, it has also become clear that early and prolonged intervention in the home, using parents as educators and other agents such as community nurses and other paramedicals, can have a significant effect upon the early development of the moderately or severely retarded. Mittler (1970) and his colleagues including Whelan (1973) and Grant, Whelan & Moores (1973) have been outstanding examples of psychologists concerned to develop such practices and to base them on sound experiment at the laboratory level as well as to try them out in an ecologically valid setting. One incidental finding of much of that work has been pointed up by the Clarkes (1977). They indicate that, with particular reference to the severely retarded, what is needed is lengthy, skilled and consequently costly help, not unskilled care-taking. This again bears particular reference to some of the main recommendations of the Jay Committee Report which in some respects seem to run counter to this.

From this rather idiosyncratic view of contributions in the past two decades from clinical psychologists in handicap it can readily be appreciated then that most have rightly divided their time between being scientists, sharp-eyed and tough-minded, and being helpers, starry eyed and soft hearted, concerned to improve the quality of life for the handicapped. There will be some who feel that the two roles cannot be happily combined and it is certainly true that the uncritical assumption of any one of them offers particular difficulties and imposes its own pressures. Nevertheless, it is unusual to find a clinical psychologist in handicap who has found the problem of moving from the role of researcher to that of the donor of a service unduly difficult. It is interesting that Haywood (1976) has stressed that psychologists should be concerned to maintain four principles in the care of the handicapped. They should be protected from both physical and psychological harm; they should be protected from invasion of privacy; they should be allowed guarantee of choice, i.e. informed consent; and finally, they should be protected from exploitation either by others or as guinea pigs in research by psychologists. In carrying out both research and clinical practice, psychologists must therefore bear these concerns in mind but at the same time they must be examined in the context of the responsibilities of professionals as scientists. These responsibilities clearly include (a) finding the best methods of treatment, education, habilitation and care; (b) encouraging good research and (c) protecting subjects from violation of any of the four principles outlined above. Finally, Haywood would suggest that we should protect the handicapped from trivial research. We must waste the time neither of our subjects nor of our colleagues. For those who are concerned to choose new areas of research, Haywood's (1976) paper can be recommended. As editor of the American Journal of Mental Deficiency he is in a strong position to advise, and several of his recommendations for what is needed in the research field are worthy of closer scrutiny.

Research is not, of course, lacking. Although the writer has chosen to illustrate the few points made from researches which could be described more as applied than fundamental, Zeaman (1974) estimated that, having counted published studies of an experimental nature in the journals available in the English literature, there was an output rate of about one every three days in the area of handicap and deficiency alone. Brooks & Baumeister (1977) have asked themselves how much greater is our understanding of mental retardation as a result of all this research activity and they make a very strong plea, based on their view of mental retardation as first and foremost a social phenomenon, for research being ecologically valid. It is not always entirely clear what these writers mean by this term since it was originally coined by Brunswick (1955,

1956). Brunswick's position followed directly from his theory that behaviour is essentially probabilistic and multiply mediated. On the receptor side, the organism is stimulated by a variety of proximal cues, having imperfect correlations with external stimuli or distal cues. He called this degree of correlation between proximal and distal cues 'ecological validity'. The proximal cues are weighted differentially in determining a response. The correlation between a given proximal cue and a response was called 'functional validity'. Brooks & Baumeister (1977), however, are more concerned with the generality of laboratory findings. Laboratory research is characterised by orderly manipulation of a small number of variables holding others constant, and by a restricted set of values of the variables manipulated. In natural, or so-called real life settings, quite different relations among the variables are likely to hold and different combinations of values may be present. It is a legitimate concern that unknown interactive effects may affect performance in such situations and one must also grant that psychologists often neglect the question of the limits of generality.

However, House (1977) in her reply to Brooks & Baumeister makes the point that even if events in nature are complex, that does not necessarily contraindicate the contolled experimental study of simpler situations. Brooks & Baumeister are in essence making a plea for research which is directly geared to an alleviation of the situation of the retardate in his actual context rather than an understanding of the processes that operate within him when he is exposed to laboratory procedures. They believe that many of the problems dogging research are related to the definition of mental retardation in terms of formal IQ. They also maintain that present techniques bear a heavy reliance on methodology that is not necessarily appropriate to the defining criteria of mental retardation as they see it and they stress the point made early in this paper that, when it comes to an individual habilitative or rehabilitative programme, the IQ is not a particularly useful bit of information.

Brooks & Baumeister make a plea for the evaluation of subject groups not just on standard IQ tests but on the basis of skills important for adapation, academic learning, language skills, motor skills and social skills and so forth. Consequently a major step in this direction would be the development of good laboratory measures that are directly reflective of these adaptive skills. As they put it, 'still another critical step in the construction of useful theories of retarded functioning is the development of meaningful taxonomies of adaptive behaviour as well as the procedures and statistics that will facilitate the description and measurement of this kind of behaviour'. They feel that in the past, psychologists have been more concerned with precise measurments than with important ones. House replies in her 1977 paper to these criticisms on the basis that, of course, IQ is, when seen as a trait, remarkably accurately measured and offers possibly a firmer criterion than some of those suggested by Brooks & Baumeister. She goes on to defend the view that retardation must be linked to hypothetical constructs such as capacities and processes but we need to show which of these capacities or processes are different in retarded and non-retarded individuals and that we need to know the general laws governing human functioning and a theory of individual differences within the general theory. As she puts it, subjects, whether retarded or not, are going to be the same subjects whether they are in the laboratory or out of it.

As with many of these theoretical debates it seems likely that the correct answer is one in which there is compromise between the two extreme points of view just as over the years the Ellis/Zigler controversy between a 'difference theory' and a motivational/developmental theory to explain moderate levels of handicap has been adjusted in the light of experience with the handicapped and persisting laboratory studies; the difference theory in fact carrying the heavier weight with the severely retarded, the motivational/developmental theory with the moderately. Nevertheless, it is important to recognise the debt we owe to clinical psychologists in handicap who are pointing up these fairly fundamental theoretical differences. There is probably no other way in which each of us, working from time to time as hard headed experimentalist and scientist and from time to time as a soft hearted carer and curer, can gather together conceptually the many strands of knowledge and endeavour that our colleagues in the field are weaving in an attempt to make some general fabric which will wear well when put to the practical test. Over the past 20 years or so the work of practising clinical psychologists in handicap has been illumined by ingenious experiment, by bold thinking and by innovative combinations of these. General psychology has certainly profited. Many of us are encouraged to believe that the handicapped themselves have lived fuller and better lives as a result, and that we are on the way at least to understanding them and helping them even more. Selective scrutiny of the better journals of research and practice in mental handicap demonstrates further efforts to add to our store of information and ideas, as well as to our knowledge of what practices should be perpetuated and examined more closely. As it was put by the Clarkes (1977) not so long ago, 'It is the task of science to reveal the way in which our biological and social pathologies can be alleviated, and it is our task as scientists to see that these findings are widely disseminated and used with profit'.

CHAPTER III

SENSORY MOTOR TRAINING

While the cynicism of the epigrammist would have us believe that a classic is a work that is frequently cited but seldom read, there can be little doubt that the beginnings of sensory motor training with the subnormal are founded in Itard's *The Wild Boy of Aveyron* (1932), in which he described his work with a feral child found in a wooded area near Paris the best part of two centuries ago. Itard set himself five main aims for his educational strategy. The first was to 'interest the wild boy in social life by rendering it more pleasant to him than the one he was leading and above all more like the life which he had just left'. Secondly, he aimed to 'awaken his nervous sensibility by the most energetic stimulation, and occasionally by intense emotion'. Thirdly, he aimed to 'extend the range of his ideas by giving him new needs and by exercising them in a social context'. Fourthly, he aimed 'to lead him to the use of speech by inducing the exercise of imitation through the imperious law of necessity'. And finally, he aimed to make him exercise 'the simplest mental operations upon the objects of his physical needs over a period of time, afterwards inducing the application of these mental processes to the objects of instruction'. By the 1840s Seguin, a student of Itard's, had demonstrated the efficacy of the latter's methods and incorporated them into a broader context so as to ameliorate the serious lack of care for the profoundly subnormal at that time. Many of Seguin's techniques were ingenious and worthy of imitation even to this day. His aim was a broader one than tends to be the case today, incorporating not just sensory motor education but extending to the realms of moral education and the training of 'willed activity'.

By the turn of the century, however, psychology and psychiatry had other preoccupations and the former in particular became obsessed with classification and measurement to the detriment of pursuing methods of training and rehabilitation. It took a more modern preoccupation with arousal and the orienting reaction whereby we have come to appreciate need for the waking brain to be exposed constantly to sensory bombardment for full efficiency, together with the growing concern among psychologists to assess the detailed aspects of cognitive function which contribute to a given overall IQ level, to reactivate an interest in training methods and in sensory-motor education in particular. It has become both easy and fashionable to set up programmes of sensory motor training in institutions dealing with the mentally subnormal, the physically disabled, the spastic and with other groups of patients requiring active rehabilitation. It is equally easy to lean on the early work of Itard, Seguin, Montessori and to support this with intuitive awareness that it must all be doing some good. One main function of this chapter is to look at more recent work which might justify such an activity and would support the legacy of earlier days in determining the day to day content of such sensory training programmes.

Those who are not handicapped tend to be preoccupied with the academically valued skills of conceptualisation, communication and conciseness. It is perhaps all too easy to forget that the earliest and, some might say, the most important skills we have learned are of a rather different category. Although our first repeated monosyllables were no doubt welcomed and reinforced by loving parents, each of us has indulged in a variety of important preliminaries such as learning to move our hands in front of our face, to follow objects with our eyes, to differentiate ourselves from our environment, to sit up, to discriminate textures, colours and shapes, to know the position of our bodies and limbs and eventually to orient ourselves in a very complex environment. Thereafter, we advance to higher level activities such as naming things and utilising concepts of number, volume and so forth. In other words, motor abilities and skills not only precede our higher cerebral activities but can be thought of as being peculiarly important in man's evolution and his attempts to control his environment. Many would agree that they are fundamental to the emergence of complex psychological processes and are a primary means of expression available to the young child.

Since considerable literature is now available indicating that motor skills are fundamental to subsequent educational endeavour, and to the development of effective cognition, it is perhaps worthwhile to digress for a moment and look at the nature of motor activity. It is, after all, one of the primary criteria for life itself and the complications involved in it have been of perennial interest. Co-ordination, speed, accuracy, beauty of movement even in walking, throwing things, handling tools and so forth, not only evoke admiration but produce responses by others to the individual carrying them out. It is equally clear that there are striking individual differences not only in the quantity of motor activity but also in its quality. In discussing problems of the handicapped it is clear that there are anatomical and physiological characteristics of the organism which will determine the extent to which motor development can occur, and in the case of many subnormals there will be fundamental difficulties of anatomy, stature and neuro-muscular co-ordination which will interfere with normal development. Moreover, emotional wellbeing will also play its part in the nature of motor development.

While much of the chapter will concern itself with the links between sensory experience and motor activity in particular, it is perhaps worth looking at the number of ways in which motor ability and motor behaviour in general can be classified. For example, motor ability and skill are often used in a confused way. In general motor ability will often be taken to be an inherent or innate characteristic, developmentally determined, whereas motor skill implies a certain amount of learning or the application of particular motor abilities to specific tasks. Most scientific studies indicate that motor skill is certainly not a unitary factor and that correlations between tests of both skills and motor abilities tend to be rather lower than between the separate parts of intelligence tests (Sloan, 1955). In general it can be taken that the level of motor ability will determine the ultimate rate and level of proficiency that can be expected in motor skills. The latter are therefore dependent not only on biological determinants but also on how well the individual learns from experience.

There is a wide acceptance of the view that the major components of motor ability include force or strength, speed and precision. The first tends to be measured by such indices as strength of grip, using a dynamometer; but there is also a more dynamic aspect of strength indicated by the capacity to propel or lift the body weight. Most studies indicate incremental changes in strength with age through adolescence and suggest that static dynamometric strength is strongly related to biological growth and constitutional factors. The increase in strength of males with age is more marked than that for females.

There is an extensive bibliography on the second of these elements, reaction time or speed of motor performance. Speed is, of course, very much a function of the intensity of the stimulus of the sense organ being stimulated and the complexity of the response required. This is one of the most widely reported variables in experimental psychology and there is an extensive literature both on normals and subnormals. The vast majority of the latter indicate that subnormals have, in general, a slower reaction time than normals and that this correlates to some extent with their IQ. There is also evidence (Ellis & Sloan, 1957) indicating greater variability among defectives than normals with respect to reaction time. Familial subnormals also tend to perform rather faster than organically damaged subjects but none of the studies indicates that IQ is related to the speed of information reception at least for subjects with no observable CNS lesions nor to cortical processes involved in initiating movement. In general, the slower reaction time of the mentally handicapped is primarily a motor or response function.

The third major component of motor ability is precision. In general, lower grade handicapped subjects demonstrate fundamentally greater difficulty in placing, turning and positioning movements in control of continuous movement and in muscular steadiness. Clark (1975) has produced data confirming this and showing correlations ranging from 0.17 in the case of steadiness, to 0.60 in the case of control of continuous movement with intelligence. However, it should be noted that some of these characteristics vary as a function of the complexity of the task required (Heath, 1942).

It is clear that biological, psychological and cultural considerations all contribute to response tendencies including motor skills. Individual variations determined by hereditary factors are easily observable since the responses of monozygotic twins clearly differ much less than the responses of bizygotic twins, siblings or relatives at further removes.

There have been attempts by, for example, Strauss & Lehtinen (1951) to provide motor performance criteria for distinguishing between exogenous and endogenous brain injured children or more generally between familial and organic groups of defectives. The differences thus obtained, however, cannot be exclusively related to genetic factors. The connection may be more indirect and it is suggested by Malpass (1963) that it is possible that many defects distinguishing these two groups, once considered to be determined by developmental anomalies, and attributed to unknown causes, may turn out to be generally determined as has been demonstrated for mongolism and phenylketonuria. Furthermore, subtle defects may be related to sex chromosomes and autosomal differences which are only now being explored for the first time, e.g. mosaicism and various trisomies. In general, though there may be some hereditary component determining the ultimate level of motor ability, for most motor skill performances, however, it is probably an interaction between genetic, developmental and stimulus reinforcement conditions which determines the ultimate level of the individual.

Establishment of linkages between specific central nervous system damage and specific motor skill performance defect have not been clearly established. In general there has been a tacit assumption when examining brain/behaviour relationships in neurologically impaired subnormals to view brain injury as a unitary variable with certain inevitable behavioural consequences (McFie, 1960), and Reitan has widely demonstrated that differential patterns and degrees of adaptive ability can be associated with specific CNS disease processes in the sites of involvement. This work, however, is not detailed enough for specific links with neurological or biological mechanisms to be established. Matthews (1961) used the Halstead-Reitan test battery on subnormals and his study suggests that motor performance of the latter group is comparable with that of recently brain injured subjects, testing at the same Wechsler IQ level (but whose pretrauma IQs were normal) on a tactual-motor task.

A great difficulty in the establishment of the linkages mentioned above derives from the different methodologies employed in studying sensory motor function, especially in defectives. The difficulties include the use of different criteria by different investigators, inadequate control of presentation conditions, administration problems in getting defectives to respond to a signal, confounding of perceptual response activities. The general view of Malpass (1963) is that it seems likely that it is in terms of response factors rather than perceptual factors that retardates suffer in comparison with normals.

It has been already indicated that there is likely to be co-variation between increases in general body growth, motor proficiency and increases in age through childhood. The general findings, reviewed by Thompson (1954) indicate that gross motor skills tend to increase with chronological age until about age 16, when there is a plateau in the curve until about age 20, followed by a minor decrease. This is true for global motor skills but not for particular skills. The developmental curves for subnormals approximate to those of normals but there is in general a delay in the demonstration of motor skills dependent on the age and IQ group considered. The analogy both for subnormals in terms of motor skills and for motor skills against cognitive development generally is clear. One thing which is clear is that there is no doubt that children designated as retarded in adolescence and adulthood, demonstrate developmental retardation in infancy. For example, Malpass (1959) reports that more than 45% of subnormal adolescents were not walking by the 16th postpartum month and 20% did not walk until after 26 months of age. 52% of retardates had not achieved bowel control and 55% had not achieved urinary control by 2 years of age, an age at which 80 to 90% of normals achieve this control.

It is also clear that as age increases through adolescence, differences between normals and retardates in gross motor skills tend to progressively increase. However, it is likely that subnormals are not stimulated to practise motor skills as much as, or as appropriately as, normals and further that they may be limited by skeletal and anatomical differences from so practising. It has been suggested by Holman (1932) and others, that initial discrepancy scores between subnormals and normals on motor and mechanical performance tasks, however, decrease with training and that this discrepancy decrease is clearly a function of greater increase in the defective scores with practice. Gordon, O'Connor & Tizard (1954) showed early on that in a study of low grade defectives a greater proportional increase in speed of performance could be expected with training when such subjects are compared to normals, even though the completion trials showed significant performance differences favouring the normals. While there is some evidence (Ammons, 1958) that normals can quickly reinstitute complex motor skills which have not been practised for up to two years, there is some doubt about how effectively subnormals can redevelop skills of this sort. However, Tizard & Loos (1954) reported that imbeciles demonstrate some retention of a learned simple motor skill. More research is necessary to clarify this point. In general, it seems safe to assume that the principles that govern most other types of learning are equally applicable to motor educability.

The work reviewed by Malpass (1963) suggests that in normal groups i.e. IQ between 90 and 110, insignificant or very low positive relationships between motor and mental ability variables are measured. However, the motor abilities reported in the relevant researches have been rather specific and no general motor factor or ability has been designated. Even fine and gross motor abilities are not necessarily related to each other so that it is not surprising that measures of motility which involve different muscle groups do not show high correspondence in studies of normal subjects.

There are, however, sex differences on measures of skill depending on strength, speed and agility, observed in the adolescent age group (Francis & Rarick, 1960). Rabin (1957) has also reported sex differences in motor proficiency of subnormals on the Lincoln-Oseretsky scale but his findings are open to some question because of separate sex norms used in standardising the scale. It seems not unlikely that the specific training given to the separate sexes, and the general social reinforcement associated with this, may produce differential motor skill performance related to sex.

However, in the case of mentally retarded subjects the correlations between IQ and motor skill tend to be substantially higher, (Distefano, Ellis & Sloan, 1958; Rabin, 1957). These correlations tend to range between 0.15 and 0.62 with many clustering around 0.4

Heath (1942) and (1953) has extensively studied the Rail Walking Test in familial and non-familial defectives and he reports that the mental test and Rail Walking performances showed lower correlations in the familial than in the non-familial subjects, 0.23 and 0.15 for familials, 0.60 and 0.57 for non-familials. However, it should be noted that these correlations in the organic group could be inflated by the necessarily lower standard deviation of test scores on both variables for the latter group.

On other measures of particular skills such as a hand steadiness test and the Minnesota Rate of Manipulation Test as used in the Distefano studies correlations ranging from 0.37 to 0.45 were reported for the institutionalised groups of defectives between the subtests and the 1937 Stanford Binet scaled scores. However, very low r's were noted between hand steadiness and mental test scores (0.16 for boys and 0.05 for girls). In summary, Malpass states 'these results suggest that correlations between measures of unitary motor skills and intelligence test scores can be expected to vary. None of the investigations demonstrates true predictive significance of mental ability from a knowledge of the motor skill or vice versa. Perhaps the best that can be stated is that scores from some of these measures of particular skills, e.g. the Heath Rail Walking Test and Minnesota Rate of Manipulation Test, correspond somewhat with Stanford Binet scaled scores for institutionalised mental defectives'.

When the Lincoln-Oseretsky scale is used, however, correlations in general for subnormals are relatively high i.e. with Stanford Binet scales. Both Rabin (1957) and Distefano et al (1958) reported significant product moment correlations between motor and mental test scores. In the case of Distefano et al 0.40 and 0.58 for institutionalised boys and girls respectively, and Malpass has also reported r's of 0.48 and 0.27 for institutionalised boys and girls. Motor performance, as measured by the Lincoln-Oseretsky, therefore is moderately related to mental ability and measured by both the WISC and the Stanford Binet.

Many of these studies have in general been with moderately retarded persons. Severely retarded people are hampered in the test situation by their general lack of responsiveness to directions, and reliability of objective studies of motor performance is difficult to achieve. In general, the clinical aetiology of mental deficiency is of some importance and a number of authorities have suggested that brain damaged subjects tend to demonstrate quantitatively and qualitatively more severe motor defects than those diagnosed as familial. It is the moderately retarded group who are most likely to be able to improve their comparatively lower motor skills by stimulation and better training methods probably over a longer period of time.

Some of the correlations between a variety of motor performances and measured intelligence reported above would seem to hint at the possibility of the former mediating the latter. This is, of course, one of the underlying assumptions behind the practice of sensory motor stimulation in the handicapped. It is crucial, however, to note that it is not simply the motor stimulation of the handicapped but the linkage of motor performance to sensory experience which is the basis of most of the early work of researchers such as Kephart (1960), Webb (1969) and Edgar, Ball, McIntyre & Shotwell (1969). Several of these will be referred to in more detail later.

In any consideration of the development of skills it is attractive to adopt, with Connolly (1969, 1970) Crossman's (1964) approach dividing performance into input, output and central processing functions, since this approach underlines the intimate connection between sensory and motor processes. In stressing the fundamental interaction between these two and that they cannot ever be thought of as being functionally independent. Connolly comments, 'An appreciation ... of the mechanisms subserving the development of sensory motor and sensory-sensory integration is essential if we are to understand the emergence of motor control, which of itself, is fundamental to the development of basic cognitive skills'. Kephart (1960) supports this vigorously and places himself well into Piaget's camp in his emphasis on the motor component of intellectual development. According to Kephart, at the earliest stages the child's information processing strategy is largely motor in nature. If his motor patterns are inadequately developed, he is literally unable meaningfully to contact and apprehend the world around him. In later stages the motor component will become subservient to the child's evolving perceptual and conceptual abilities, but there is little doubt that Kephart would take the view, even if it seems an over-emphatic one, that initially intellectual deficiencies tend to amount to a disrupted and undeveloped motor system.

Kephart has developed an intensive perceptual motor programme based on basic motor patterns which he considers to be important for the future learning of specific skills. These motor patterns are:

(1) Balance and posture. Through this movement pattern the child gains a knowledge of gravity and his relationship to it. From this there develops an understanding of spatial relationships, such as right left, up down, front back and so forth.

(2) Locomotion. Locomotion skills move the child through space helping him to learn about the relationships of objects in space to himself and

helping him to learn about the relationships between these objects in space themselves.

(3) Receipt and propulsion. The child learns to make contact with moving objects and to impart movement to objects.

(4) Contact. The child learns about reaching, grasping and releasing objects, learning also about form, shape and size.

It is Kephart's view that mastery of these basic movement patterns allows the development of specific skills and that with increased perceptual motor control the child will exhibit enhanced intellectual performance. While there are strong resemblances to Piagetian thinking in this, Kephart has had his share of critics who have taken the view that while he seems to have some clinical success with an adoption of these principles his work requires further experimental verification. Webb (1969) has also developed a parallel system aimed at improving level of awareness, movement, manipulation of the environment and posture and locomotion which will be referred to later.

If Kephart acknowledges the influence of Piaget (1952), he has also drawn on a neuro-psychological model of Hebb (1949) through which he accounts for the disruption that occurs in the learning process of disabled learners. Some of the theoretical rationale for treatment strategies comes from Hebb but in fact many of his practical remediation activities reflect much more the influence of Madame Montessori (1964) who in turn developed her ideas and practices from those of Seguin, the grandfather of all sensory motor training.

Kephart and Webb share to some extent the influence of Henry Head (1925), his notion of the development of body schemata, and his preoccupation with the view that in the developmental task of becoming aware of his own body the infant is concerned with the importance of stimuli from within the skin i.e. those of proprioceptive origin. Some of the most important pieces of information are transmitted from the vestibular organs of the inner ear and from kinaesthetic receptors in muscles and tendons. Ball (1971) has developed an interesting and useful, if slightly lengthy, analogy from space flight which, he maintains, is an appropriate phenomenological frame of reference for Kephart's theory.

> Imagine yourself going to sleep at home. Waking, you find you are sealed in some type of enclosure. (It is, in fact, a space vehicle orbiting the earth, but you are not aware of this). Inside, it is pitch-black; you cannot see outside and your condition is one of weightlessness. The only moveable object within the cockpit-enclosure is a control stick which, unknown to you, activates elevators and ailerons—control surfaces that cause the vehicle to tilt, or to rise and fall, when moving through the atmosphere. You are, however, not *in* the atmosphere so control surfaces have no effect. Further, due to your weightlessness, you are unaware that the craft is spinning slowly on its axis. You manipulate the control stick, uselessly, but there is no correlation between this voluntary movement and other bodily sensations.

In general, you do not know the nature or the function of your enclosure. The problem is to determine what is happening to you and whether or not you have any control over the situation.

While these circumstances depict a claustrophobic nightmare, they also suggest the problems involved at the earliest stages of learning. Clearly, the first piece of required information is that of a *correlation* between voluntary activity and resultant feedback. Such learning, however, cannot occur in orbit. For the necessary correlations to occur we must add the all-important factor, *gravity*. This could be accomplished by slowing the speed of the vehicle until it went out of orbit and entered the earth's atmosphere. Assume that you, as the unknowing "pilot", were again unaware of such a change. For lack of anything else to do, you continue moving the single control, but this time a movement is correlated with a unique set of bodily sensations. Thus, you move the stick to the right and you experience vestibular stimulation and increased tactual feedback from the right side of your body. Further, there is a felt discrepancy between your right and left sides. You move the stick to the right, then forward and back. Each movement, in turn, is associated with a distinctive pattern of bodily sensation. As you learn this series of correlations between kinaesthetic patterns incidental to voluntary movement of the control stick and passively experienced bodily sensations caused by resulting changes in position, you develop a frame of reference within the darkened cockpit. At this point you are still helpless and unable meaningfully to guide the craft. Yet the time is not wasted because you are establishing a *system of coordinates* into which you can potentially plug other data as they become available. As your gliding craft gradually loses altitude, the opaque covering over the cockpit disappears and you find yourself peering through a translucent, but not transparent, window. You can discern only the horizon line—that demarcation between the darkened earth and the sky above. At this point, you do not know that it is actually the horizon or that you are viewing anything "out there". It is just an ill-defined boundary, lacking details. Now, however, you have a source of visual input which can be fed into your previously established kinaesthetic-tactual-vestibular coordinate system. You push the control stick forward and the horizon line floats upward, you push it to the left and it tilts; you repeat these actions, always with the same result. You are now *matching* visual data against prior kinaesthetic, tactual and vestibular data. Your experiential frame of reference has expanded. Thus, visual input is correlated with previously integrated kinaesthetic, tactual and vestibular input—the movement of the line acquires meaning in terms of a bodily frame of reference; it tilts when you tilt.

At this point, the translucent windshield is replaced with a semi-transparent one. You become aware that there *is* an "out there". In addition to the horizon gradient or line of demarcation, new gradients of lightness and darkness appear corresponding to land and water masses. However, you have not identified them as such. Nor, for that matter, are you even aware that you are circling the earth. Nonetheless, as you continue to orbit you detect a certain regularity in the *succession* of gradients, and as you lose altitude the gradients become more *distinct*. You conclude that you are, in fact, orbiting a planet with irregular surfaces. If the gradients represent differences in elevation, the craft would have to be carefully manoeuvred to effect a safe landing, but you lack sufficient detail to distinguish between a mountain and a plain as prospective locations for such a landing.

Finally, the semi-transparent window is replaced by a fully transparent one and you can, for the first time, see details of the terrain below. You must reappraise your situation based on the *relationships* between such details. Effecting a safe landing is not merely a matter of finding level ground, but rather level ground of adequate length. Further, the accessibility of level ground must be considered in relation to other features of the terrain; for example, a valley nestled within a mountain range may be sufficiently long but inaccessible. At this point your visual frame of reference is expanded to its full extent. Yet, although it has become predominant, it is still operating in correlation with and in ultimate reference to the originally established proprioceptive coordinate system.

From this point on, with the exception of the final descent, you can continue to view the surface below. However, your focus of attention shifts to making calculations related to a strategy for getting the craft safely down; calculations such as estimations of velocity, possibilities for last-minute corrections in gliding path, etc. While based on the outer scene, these abstract manipulations transcend it; that is, they relate to future possibilities, rather than to the immediate realities of sensory input.

Other experimental approaches have pointed up how deprivation of the right sorts of sensory and motor experience can lead to a degradation of performance on perceptual motor tasks (Freedman, 1961). Riesen (1958) has shown also that the young of primates and some other mammals tend to fail to develop normal visually guided behaviour when they are deprived of visual contact with a stimulating environment. Clearly, sensory motor control can therefore be adversely affected by poverty of input. Other experiments by Held & Hein (1958) and Held & Schlank (1959) have investigated different conditions (no movement, passive movement and active movement) and found that only active movement, i.e. movements controlled by the subject resulted in adaptation. Passive movement when the subject's limb was moved by an experimenter did not result in adaptation despite the fact that the views of the hand and the motion were identical. The results of these studies suggest that the connection between motor output and sensory input which is lacking in the passive movement condition is crucial for adaptation to take place.

One of the best known experiments illustrating the adverse effect of sensory motor deprivation of a certain type of motor development has been carried out by Held & Hein (1963) who investigated the importance of movement-produced stimulation in the development of visually guided behaviour in kittens. They used an apparatus in which the gross movements of a kitten, moving as it normally would, were transmitted directly to another kitten carried in a gondola.

By using this apparatus they were enabled to investigate the effects of active and passive transport in a limited area where the visual stimulation was exactly identical for both animals. The kittens were reared in darkness until the one chosen as the active member of each pair was strong enough to move its partner in the swinging gondola somewhere around 8 to 12 weeks old. The animals were in the apparatus for three hours each day. The apparatus itself provided a simple striped pattern around the walls of the arena which was used. When not in the apparatus the kittens were kept in complete darkness and after approximately 30 hours of such experience the active member of each pair showed normal behaviour on a range of visually guided tasks. For example, it blinked at the approach of an object, made placing movements when carried down towards a surface and avoided the steep side of a visual cliff. On the other hand the passively moved kitten failed to show these behaviours, developing these only gradually after it had been given sufficient time in which to move around actively in a normal environment.

The same authors have also looked at the importance for an animal of viewing its own actively moving limbs if it is to make accurate visual placing responses. Following a special rearing procedure Held & Hein (1967) were able to show with a refined testing technique that kittens may extend their fore limbs on approach to a surface but they were unable to guide their limb towards a particular object. Experimental kittens were reared without the sight of their limbs by making use of an opaque plastic collar which was placed around their necks. By doing this the only restriction placed on the kitten was the prevention of visual experience of its own limbs since it could see everything else. No restrictions were placed on their movements or on visual stimulation. The experimenters measured the effects of the experimental procedure by evaluating the kitten's placing response by holding the animal with its four legs free and moving it down towards an interrupted surface of castellated pattern. All the animals tended to produce a placing response when this was carried out but whereas the controls contacted the surface on 95% of the trials the experimental animals showed an accurately guided placing response on less than 50% of the trials. Similarly, when the experimental kittens were tested with a ball dangling on a string they oriented normally towards it with head and eyes but were quite inaccurate at striking it with their paws. As in the previous experiment when the collars were removed and the experimental animals had about 18 hours of normal movement in visual experience they recovered to the level of the control animals.

Something of the same findings hold good for monkeys. Held & Bauer (1967) tested this by rearing a monkey long enough for maturation to enable it to carry out visually guided reaching but rearing it in such a way that the apparatus prevented it from having visual experience of its body. Some 35 days after birth one hand was exposed to view and naturally the monkey looked long and hard at it. However, visually guided reaching with this limb was significantly poor but it improved very quickly over ten hours. The previously unexposed limb, however, showed little or no improvement until eventually four months after the experiment the experimental monkeys developed visually guided behaviours bilaterally and were then indistinguishable from the normally reared controls. It is clear therefore, that the early experience of watching the moving parts of our bodies provides the information which is necessary for matching the visual orientation to a target with the limb movement for reaching it.

Connolly (1969) has pointed out that so far as humans are concerned both Gesell & Amatruda (1947) and Piaget (1952) have studied the emergence of prehension and visually directed reaching in infants but Gesell's theoretical position of seeing this as a maturation led him to be more interested in the establishment of norms than to a concern with the morphology of the developing response system. Piaget watched this development in his own children but being concerned with cognition and the establishment of mental structures his data is more limited. White, Castle & Held (1964) have described the course of the development of visually directed reaching in the human infant. They found that an infant will swipe at an object at about 2½ months, at 3 months the hands will be brought to the midline and clasped and at about a month and a half later the baby will rapidly lift his hand from the visual field to the object and as it approaches the object it will open in anticipation of touching it. In later work White & Held (1967) investigated the effects of experimental modifications of the development of visual motor behaviour in infants. Looking first at infants born and reared in an institution because of inadequate family conditions they were able to show favourable effects on visual exploratory behaviour and reaching, attributable to extra 20 minutes handling per day. In view of the animal studies reported earlier, these authors then attempted to investigate the effects of enrichment in visual stimulation coupled with increasing the likelihood of movement and did so by placing the babies in a prone position with the sides of the cot lowered and what they call stabiles consisting of contrasting colours and shapes were suspended against the dull white ground to increase the visual stimulation. One effect of this treatment was to set back hand regard and swiping but what they call prehension or grasping and reaching was advanced by 45 days.

The third investigation of these authors combined their previous efforts in that between the sixth and thirty-sixth day the infants were given extra handling and this was followed between days 37 and 68 with exposure to design stimuli mounted on the crib in the form of two nipples attached to bright red and white backgrounds positioned on either side of the crib about 6 to 7 inches from the corneal surface of the infants' eyes. These objects elicited maximum attention from a 6 to 8 week old infant and it was thought that they might have the effect of orienting the infant towards his hands. From day 68 to day 124 the stabiles were suspended over the cot and the results of this study indicated a striking increase in the rate of development of visually directed reaching. Hand regard and swiping appeared at 46 days, prehension developed at less than 3 months and visual attention was increased.

Supporting these previous experiments with both animals and humans is another reported by Minden (1972) who carried out experiments with 16 rats randomly assigned to each of three experimental conditions. Six were on what he called forced activity, five on voluntary activity and five on restricted condition. Briefly, rats in the forced activity group were placed individually into a training apparatus in which they had to run on a moving belt for 15 minutes per day for 24 days. The voluntary activity occurred in a stationary training apparatus where subjects were allowed to run and explore freely but were not compelled to activity, whereas the restricted subjects were confined to relatively small cages where negligible activity was possible. The criterion measure was ability to swim a water maze with few errors and it was apparent that forced activity subjects made significantly fewer errors in this than the voluntarily active subjects who in turn made fewer errors than the restricted ones. There was also a significant difference in the latency between the groups with the same ranking. This work by Minden (1972) replicates experiments by Hebb (1949) who was able to show that rats reared as pets in a household were superior to cage-raised rats in problem solving as measured by the Hebb-Williams maze. There have been subsequent replications of these researches all showing a higher level of problem solving in animals who are given more complex motor and visual environment. It should be noted, however, that Hebb's (1949) conception of the development of cell assemblies and phase sequences emphasises perceptual experience rather than motor experience, whereas other theories, such as those of Osgood (1953) and Piaget (1952) have argued that motor behaviour structures the central process and that sensory motor experiences are the fundamental building blocks for more complex perceptual and cognitive development.

Replication in a systematic way of the early studies of the effects of infantile experience on problem-solving ability measured by the Hebb-Williams Intelligence Test for rats was carried out by Hymovitch in 1952. The intelligent behaviour of rats brought up in an open environment was compared with that of rats brought up in cages with wooden walls which limited their visual experience but did not eliminate pattern vision. The free environment rats showed a substantial superiority over the others but Hymovitch (1952) found, nevertheless, that animals reared in mesh cages placed within the free environment performed indistinguishably from those reared in a free environment. He argued that so far as the mesh cages restricted the motor experience of these animals but did not prevent their seeing the wooden and metal structures placed outside their cages it must be a perceptual experience rather than a motor experience that was important in the establishment of the central processes which facilitate problem solving. Minden (1972) takes the view that such a conclusion may have been premature and he quotes work by Forgays & Forgays (1952) which found that animals allowed motor experience in free environment were superior in problem solving to any group reared in mesh cages. This superiority was found regardless of the nature of the environment surrounding the mesh cages and since this superiority was substantial it appeared that motor experience may be an important factor in the development of intelligence. This study has been replicated on at least four other occasions with similar results, and is, of course, consistent with the work of Held & Hein quoted earlier. In general, therefore, the development of co-ordinated behaviour demands early variation in visual stimulation which will be most effective when it is concurrent with self-produced movement.

These experiments suggest quite clearly that self-controlled movement plays an important and even critical role in the young animal's or infant's development. Again this seems to indicate a correlation between motor output and sensory feedback since during the course of a number of movements the nervous system may take account of the internally initiated efferent signals to the skeletal musculature together with their concurrent visual feedback. As Connolly (1969) remarks, 'Within the limits of precision permitted by the transfer of information in the neuro-muscular system, the one to one relationship between movement and its sensory feedback allows the system to establish and store correlated information'.

This preoccupation with the emergence and development of sensory motor control as a simple skill is deliberate since the latter tends to imply guidance, goal directedness and a serial ordering of behaviour. As Connolly remarks, it relates also to an individual's ability to select for himself specific sources of information, to process such information and to direct his attention as in problem solving. Abercrombie (1968) has argued that impairments in perceptual motor functioning are likely to have effects on a wide range of behaviours which might emerge as an apparent lowering of intelligence both of a verbal and performance sort. Moreover it has led inevitably to the question that if insufficient motor learning experiences tend to retard motor development, can the provision of special training accelerate motor learning in those in whom it has not so far occurred? It is the earnest belief of many who indulge in sensory motor training with, for example, spastics, the mentally subnormal, hemiplegics and socially and physically deprived children that it can.

Many of the difficulties in the evaluation of such training programmes, however, derive from the fact that they frequently seek too generalised a goal or attempt to measure the effects along too broad a spectrum of performance. A second difficulty is that intrusive but frequently poorly validated and often non-univocal constructs like body image tend to be introduced as intervening variables affected by such programmes. For example, the concept of laterality as an aspect of body image has been considered to be fairly critical in a motor development hypothesis to explain aspects of school achievement but results have been far from unequivocal. O'Connor (1969) compared the effects of a traditional physical education programme and physical activities in the form suggested by Kephart (1960) on motor, perceptual and academic achievement of first grade school children and he reported in favour of the Kephart method only for measures of motor ability and internal lateral awareness. No signficant differences were found between the two methods on measures of academic achievement, external lateral awareness, lateral preference or ability to draw geometric figures.

Neil O'Connor (1966) has stressed how a number of studies of different types suggest that one of the main difficulties of the mentally handicapped is in initial learning. They do not seem able to select the appropriate cue, to attend to the aspect or dimension at issue. Once they have learned skills to overcome this, learning can be fairly rapid and retention better. It can be added that one of the best ways of cueing a young child, and one might suppose a mental defective, is through his own movements or the movements of those in his immediate environment. As has already been stressed the child's development has been noted to start with the proximate senses. He has to touch and manipulate before he can develop later to a purely distant perception which is usually visual. There is a most interesting paper by Denner & Cashdan (1967) who showed that children remembered solid shapes better after manipulating them than when they had seen them. When, however, the manipulated shape was enclosed in a clear perspex sphere it was remembered as well after handling as if it had actually been manipulated. The authors suggest that the important factor is the amount of activity exerted by the child and not the particular sensory channel employed.

It is perhaps the case with most sensory training programmes that the originators are concerned to generate a variety of activities on the part of the subjects so that these when suitably harnessed to cognitive development in general and especially to language advancement in particular will form a basis for a development of higher order cognitive activities. Maria Montessori was expressing this rather generalised approach when she remarked that 'experiences seem to be taken in through the senses, and the child works out meaning through his activity ... Learning requires concentration, and the only way a child can concentrate is by fixing his attention on a task he is performing with his hands ... When we "train" the senses, we are not trying to make a child see better, we are helping him to know what he sees'.

Related to the work of O'Connor, Hill et al (1967) investigated the effects of a systematic programme of exercises on the development of retarded children's awareness of right/left directionality. These workers concluded that programmes for training retarded children should include activities which give them many experiences in orientating their attention to the position of their own bodies in space relative to that of other objects as well as directing children to make responses with specified body parts. Tansley (1968) has repeated this message in reporting on the education of children whose difficulties lie in the areas of abnormal neurological development, perceptual disturbances or language dysfunction. Training at Tansley's school is given in such things as hand/eye coordination, form perception, visual discrimination, movement training of both a specific and a more generalised nature, the latter being directed mainly at the improvement of the child's body image. Tansley reports encouraging and quite spectacular results in the general cognitive development of children following such a programme.

Perhaps the best known critical study of the results of a Kephart type sensory motor training programme is that by Edgar, Ball, McIntyre & Shotwell (1969) which investigated the relationship between such a training course and adaptive behaviour. The subjects in this study were 22 five or six year old institutionalised moderately and severely retarded children. The 11 experimental subjects received intensive training activities for 15 to 20 minutes a day, four days a week. Control subjects were also seen for the same period each day and the same number of days per week. In the control group an attempt was made to control for possible extraneous factors such as the attention given to the experimental group by using such activities as finger painting, puzzles, listening to music, and looking at books. Mental age increases (estimated from Gesell raw scores) for the experimental and control groups were 7.7 and 1.9 months respectively over an 8 month period. Both control and experimental subjects showed significant increases in language and personal social subskills. In a further study, Ball & Edgar (1967) demonstrated a significant increase in what they called 'generalised body image development' for a group of 30 normal kindergarten children who underwent 3½ months of sensory motor training.

In a later paper by Maloney, Ball & Edgar (1970), however, a number of criticisms of these prior studies were made and the authors went on to seek to provide a more critical test of certain theoretical and practical aspects of sensory motor training. They predicted in particular that subjects given sensory motor training would demonstrate significant improvements in finger localisation after a period of specific training. They aimed to control the effects of any incidental attention to the subjects which accrued from the sensory motor training, by arranging that those not undergoing sensory motor training would have an equivalent and similar type of non-specific attention paid to them, predicting further that there would be no significant differences attributable to such attention. They were, in fact, able to show that all generalised effects of sensory motor training were not due simply to increased attention, but the study failed to support the hypothesis that generalisation from sensory motor training would occur in finger localisation after a period of specific finger training. The experimenters did yield that there appeared to be improvement in generalised body image development although they could see difficulties, as indeed many critics can, in the operational determination of body image and indeed the full meaning of the concept.

Subsequently, Morrison & Pothier (1972) tested the differential effects of two different sensory motor programmes on groups of mentally retarded children using the Denver Developmental Screening Test to assess performance before and after. Their work showed that the experimental children made significantly greater increments over the interval of training in gross motor, language and full scale scores than did the control children, and they point out further that the failure of the sensory motor training group to demonstrate a significant effect in fine motor skills is explicable in terms of Kephart's theory. His view is that perceptual motor skills progress from gross to finer perceptual motor coordination.

Webb (1969) has also developed a parallel system aimed at improving (1) level of awareness, (2) movement, (3) manipulation of the environment and (4) posture and locomotion. It is her view that profoundly retarded subjects tend to present gross underdevelopment in these general areas of behaviour. So far as the first is concerned, children may be so inert that they give no apparent response to sensory stimuli and even to withdraw actively into autistic shells. This is likely, in her view, to disrupt the normal development of recognising pleasant and unpleasant stimuli, remembering past exposures to them and exercising discrimination in anticipating or avoiding future contacts with them. The child, therefore, does not respond selectively, and intentionality becomes impossible for such retarded subjects. Secondly, the disturbance in arousal level of that kind is often associated with impairment of total body movement. Alternatively, youngsters may be hyperactive and move constantly. It is Webb's view that *both* conditions interfere with basic motor reflexes and the later integration of motor effectors with multiple sensory inputs. The normal cephalo-caudal developmental pattern is disrupted so that the retarded child does not develop evenly the gross movements which are used by normal youngsters in making progressively more adequate adjustments to the sensory stimuli received. So far as manipulation of the environment is concerned, both of the above difficulties make it much more difficult for the retardate to gain satisfaction of both physical and emotional needs by altering his physical and social environments. Fine muscle group coordination, particularly hand/eye, is not properly developed in a way which enables the child to cope with physical objects and to interact with people effectively. Finally, posture and locomotion difficulties in which the retardate is competing against gravity lead severely retarded individuals to modify their posture to a degree which may be extreme so that they both contort their trunks and limbs into inefficient shapes and have unstable upright positions from which movements through space can originate and at which movements can terminate. Consequently, knowledge of directionality and laterality are poorly learned through motor experience because the subject does not commence from a secure base in a literal sense. Similarly his incapacity effectively to explore boundaries of personal and physical space around him is undermined. The rationale for training techniques which Webb develops is based on these four characteristic difficulties, the goal of sensory motor training in her view being to 'promote the development of single attentional and motor reactions to discrete stimuli, and the integration of these simple responses into multiple sensory motor units which cut across the four behaviour areas'.

In her paper, Ruth Webb goes on to outline how 32 profoundly retarded institutionalised children with some degree of encephalopathy were given sensory motor training based on these general principles for up to ten months. She has developed rating scales for measuring the amount of treatment given and the response to it but the detailed effects of the programme are not easy to evaluate since she makes the general point that clinical analysis of changes between pre- and post-treatment behaviours tended to be more meaningful than statistical comparisons because of the dissimilarity between the measuring instruments that she used. In general there was no doubt that many of the children showed significant motor and sensory development, but the study lacked controls where either passivity replaced the sensory training programme or where an alternative activity programme was allowed. It is perhaps significant that more than half the subjects showed improvements in awareness and arousal and in behaviours deriving from this.

There have been a number of studies on the effects of different kinds of sensory motor training on retardates of different age groups recently (Chasey & Wyrick, 1971; Chasey, Swartz & Chasey, 1974; Maloney, Ball & Edgar, 1970; Kerr, McKerracher & Neufeld, 1973; Morrison & Pothier, 1972) but all of these, although being strongly suggestive of the importance to retardates of some form of sensory motor training are bedevilled by a whole variety of methodological errors. For example, many studies lack effective controls as mentioned above. Secondly, several use test techniques which are poorly validated and/or have low reliability. Very few have exactly comparable techniques of training described and frequently have inadequate descriptions of the experimental populations used. Thirdly, the criterion measures tend to vary widely from single tests of 'body image development' to the Lincoln-Oseretsky Scale Scores of motor proficiency or to specific apparatus test scores after the Fleishman (1964) model. Finally, the theoretical underpinning of many of the views put forward is scanty or negligible and while this would not be a serious criticism so long as pragmatic evaluation of the results showed significant and marked individual changes in some subjects, it is still more likely that significant advance will be made if procedures stem from an agreed theoretical position rather than being empirically evaluated, piecemeal, by this or that researcher.

This battlefield is reviewed in three recent papers in the American Journal of Mental Deficiency which illustrate nicely many of these points. The first paper is an experimental evaluation of sensory motor patterning used with mentally retarded children by Neman, Roos, McCann, Menolascino & Heal (1974). This team of psychologists from the American National Association for Retarded Citizens carried out a programme of sensory motor patterning on 66 institutionalised mentally retarded children and adolescents. Their programme of sensory motor training was, however, very specific and owed a great deal to the Doman-Delecato regimens from the Institute for the Achievement of Human Potential in Philadelphia. A general statement of these principles may be found in Le Winn, Doman, Delacato, Doman, Spitz & Thomas (1966) but serious criticisms have been presented and their general theoretical position and practical techniques have been very rigorously discredited in a critical paper by Cohen, Birch & Taft (1970) and also by Freeman (1967). This is not to say that other sensory motor programmes have been devoid of criticism. Hammill (1972) and Goodman & Hamill (1973), have also been critical of the Frostig, Kephart and Getman procedures as well as the Doman-Delacato programmes. However, there has always been ground for doubt about both the critical and the positive reviews in that very often the criterion measures have been open to a good deal of debate as Halliwell & Solan (1973) have pointed out and there are a number of other reasons for the conflicting results which are seen from study to study.

The Neman et al paper (1975) randomly assigned their 66 subjects to each of three groups, the first being an experimental (1) group which received a programme of mobility exercises including patterning, creeping and crawling, visual motor trailing and sensory stimulation exercises. The second experimental (2) group received a programme of physical activity, personal attention and the same sensory stimulation programme given to the first group, and (3) group was a passive control group which provided baseline measures but which received no additional programming as part of the study. In general, experimental (1) group subjects improved more than subjects in the other groups in visual reception, programme related measures of mobility and language ability. Intellectual functioning did not appear to be enhanced by the procedures, at least during the active phase of the project. The experimenters go on to discuss the results, particularly in relation to previous negative results, but are immediately set upon by Zigler & Seitz (1975) who presented a seriously damaging critique of the Neman et al (1974) paper.

It is probably not too much to say that the paper by Zigler & Seitz is one which should be thoroughly perused by all those who must assess both undergraduate and post-graduate research in psychology, since it effectively impresses on the reader a number of fundamental precepts which could well do with framing in any researcher's study. In brief, Zigler & Seitz (1975) deal with shortcomings of the previous paper in terms of (1) problems with the theoretical rationale underlying the treatment being assessed, (2) subject selection, (3) procedure, (4) analyses and (5) interpretations. Apart from that they slate the previous paper for premature publication, the use of unsuitable prose style and an attempt at popularisation which does less than justice to the observed data. The only point on which the critics concur with the original authors is that further evaluation of the sensory motor training treatment is needed and that the most appropriate evaluation would involve comparing the outcome of this treatment with a variety of other treatments that are or could be employed to enhance the development of retarded people.

Neman (1975) has since returned to the fray with a spirited defence of the original paper by himself and his colleagues but yields on a number of issues to Zigler & Seitz. All of these papers combine to illustrate both the current needs for research in sensory motor training and the extreme difficulties of carrying this out in a way which is experimentally impeccable and socially useful.

Among some of the precepts for sensory motor trainers which might be derived from that series of papers would be included the crucial need to use appropriate subjects representing as broad a spectrum as possible of the subnormal population so that generalisation from the particular research study is feasible. Any detailed programme which was prejudiced by tying it to a hopelessly limited sub-sample of the retarded population would be largely a waste of time since generalisability would be extremely limited. Secondly, it becomes increasingly apparent that a large number of dependent measures must be adopted. If only a few are used it may well be that those chosen may fail to reflect a real change or difference in subjects, especially if those chosen show high intercorrelations. However, it is important that dependent measures must have strong theoretical relevance: otherwise, by chance alone, some dependent variables may show significant change which could be entirely misleading. Thirdly, it seems apparent that most sensory motor programmes must have sufficient time given to them. The evidence of the literature would suggest that six months to a year is the minimum period for significant gains to be noted in most retardates, and research indicates that programmes run for a shorter time provide at best equivocal and at worst misleading results. Fourthly, there is a troubled issue in that many programmes which have used skilled personnel to see them through have tended to show, on the whole, better results than those using normal staffs or uninformed, even non-indoctrinated staff. Ethically, it would seem that there should be every encouragment to use such indoctrinated staff with the programme provided that those staff running alternative and controlled programmes are equally committed to their own techniques and approaches. The more difficult issue is how far training should be developed as a technique applied broadly to 20, 30 or more retardates and how far it should be tailored to the individual case with quite tightly defined and relatively limited individual goals. The contemporary climate of opinion in psychometrics and in psychological theory might certainly suggest that the latter, rather than the former procedure, is to be preferred and there is no doubt that the anecdotal evidence of Victor vindicates Itard's approach along these lines. On the other hand, such individualised training or treatment, sensory motor or otherwise, is expensive of personnel and time and becomes extremely difficult to validate as a general method.

For those who are interested in the content of such sensory motor training it will be clear that while there is a hierarchy of perceptual motor coordinations from gross to fine, at the same time subskills involving the establishment of laterality, perceptual motor match, directionality, movement patterns and the serial ordering of movements are significant subskills to be mastered. Moreover, tactual/kinaesthetic linkages, visual/auditory linkages, form perception and differentiation and eventually classification and concept formation tasks must all play their part in a systematic training programme along with attempts to improve posture, locomotion and manipulation of the environment. Ruth Webb (1969) has outlined specific items in a programme which hopefully would take into account all these variables. Other ideas for activities in a programme can be derived from testing instruments such as the Purdue Perceptual Motor Survey (Roach & Kephart, 1966), and Morrison & Pothier (1972) outline a detailed programme content in a second document available in conjunction with their earlier quoted paper.

Many of the exercises and activities subsumed under schemes such as these include music and movement regimes which can be carried out with groups of from 2 to 50 patients at a time, which can be subdivided so that one group of patients is involved sedentarily on manipulation, textural appreciation and sorting tasks with form boards, jigsaws, clay, plasticine, water, sand and boards containing different types of cloth or substance, while others are more actively involved in ball games, formal marching, with or without rhythmical or musical accompaniments, carrying out tasks in response to a mirror image against a full length mirror so that they are getting visual motor matching, either by looking at a mirror or by copying the movements of an instructor. A sense of weight and kinaesthetic activity can be given by using a soft environment such as a large air mattress, huge rubber balls, trampolines, hanging on ropes, crossbars, swinging or, at the simplest, passive or active rolling on soft mats. Laterality exercises which have proved valuable include the use of metre half inch dowelling rods which can be held in two hands simultaneously or by one hand on demand and which can be placed in a variety of positions in response to an instructor or model. Ball games and games with bean bags and hoops can be used to inculcate a sense of the serial order of activities and no opportunity should be lost to utilise verbal mediation of behaviour as a supportive technique.

Many team games can be utilised to establish discriminatory reactions whereby the subject responds to his or her name or obeys simple verbal commands to elicit actions other than those being generated in the rest of the group. Holding, grasping and throwing objects can start with passing a bean bag or a ball from one hand to the other, then from one hand of one subject to the hand of another subject a foot away and gradually extending the distance until a group of subjects round the instructor are sequentially receiving a thrown tennis ball, medicine ball, balloon or other object.

Textural matching games can be played by blindfolding subjects and asking them to discriminate an object of specific texture by touch from a board containing different textures such as small squares of different grades of sandpaper, woodbark, corduroy, silk and a variety of cloths or other substances, e.g. corrugated paper or glass. So far as visual-motor matching is concerned the placing of form boards and jigsaw components plays a large part in training for this and other games such as hoopla and limited forms of darts or quoits similarly contribute to such activities. The more gross postural developments required can sometimes be best achieved by formal walking, marching and dancing routines either individually or with a partner, progressing to tasks such as walking along a bench, pot walking, obstacle races demanding maximal postural and textural variety and eventually to Heath rail walking. It is interesting to note in passing that rail walking test performance was found in studies by O'Connor & Tizard (1951) and by Tizard, O'Connor & Crawford (1950) to contribute largely to the prediction of work success. Its correlation with work ratings was 0.44 and when combined with the score on a body sway test the multiple correlation coefficient was 0.52. It was found, however, that the Heath Rail Walking Test, as was noted earlier in the chapter, also differentiated between not only normals and retardates but between endogenous and exogenous retardates.

Later developments of gross locomotor coordination may involve the use of dummy steps with a handrail on one side so that subjects are taught to go up a few stairs, first holding on with the right hand and then by reversing the direction of travel holding on with the left hand and then subsequently without hand support. Similarly, fine coordination and dexterity can be developed by using large sets of nuts and bolts for screwing and unscrewing movements and discrimination of sizes and colours can be incorporated in a programme by giving sorting tasks with tins, blocks, hanks of wool, pieces of cloth and so forth. Threading activities using perforated hardboard and courlene or nylon twine can start off as a simple manipulation but be made more complex by inviting the subject to copy patterns and can lead on to more refined work with canvas and cross-stitching. In short, the content of such programmes is limited only by the ingenuity of the operator but it is important that they are not left to run on their own and instructors need to be thoroughly primed in the necessity for gauging first of all the appropriate levels of performance fitted to given subjects, to ensuring that sufficient overlearning occurs, and that over large increments of difficulty are not introduced.

Finally, while the evidence adduced in this paper would appear in general principle to warrant the maintenance of such programmes with severe retardates and would suggest that there is a good deal of generalisability of learning from specific sensory motor training programmes to wider aspects of physical development and cognitive growth, and consequently that Kephart's view of cognitive development being based on perceptual motor skills is thereby substantiated, there remains a dearth of work reporting subsequent *higher cognitive performance* attributable to sensory motor programmes of the type described. Sensory motor training will produce sensory motor progress. Motor training will produce motor progress. It may well be that the methodological problem of testing cognitive growth independent of sensory motor skills has dogged the experimental validation of Roach & Kephart's hypothesis. In other words, do subjects who were hitherto untestable because they had neither the discrimination skill nor the motor skill to respond to a test situation simply become more testable rather than more able because they have had sensory motor training; or do they develop cognitively in a more general way so that tests do in fact elicit evidence of general intellectual growth? The comparative studies quoted earlier are probably more persuasive in favour of the latter view rather than that subjects who have had sensory motor training are simply being enabled to express cognitive skills that have always been there but were previously inexpressible.

It is certainly true that if longitudinal development of individuals within a species in any way recapitulates a phylogenetic pattern, then sensory motor and perceptual skills clearly form the foundation for higher nervous activity and eventually the acquisition and use of symbolic reasoning and speech. In applying a programme of sensory motor training to the mentally subnormal there is no doubt that we are going a long way back along this developmental route. The evidence is now accumulating, however, that this is a justifiable procedure which in one form or another has been recognised by remedial teachers in other spheres for many a long day. It is almost ironic that we non-subnormals have to remind ourselves from time to time that even after a full armamentarium of concepts, symbolic skills and verbalisation capacities have been developed, these can still only be utilised by dint of motor performance at a skeletal level. Cyril Burt's enormous capacity for analysis and clarity in this thinking led him as early as 1937 first to express this now obvious fact: 'It is a truism in psychology that the mechanism of the mind stands on a sensory motor basis. The world outside can stimulate the mind only through one of the senses; and, in return, all that the greatest intellect can do is to contract a set of muscles and move a set of bony levers. The end product of every mental process is simply a muscular reaction'. The essential rationale of sensory motor training of the subnormal is that it is also the starting point.

CHAPTER IV

INSTITUTIONS AND THE PSYCHOLOGIST

Introduction

With the rapid emergence of the principles of normalisation of the mentally handicapped (Nirje, 1969, 1970) institutions have become something of a dirty word in the literature of handicap. It is not hard to see why this has happened. Throughout the UK the legacy of the past 100 years is evident in the form of large, sometimes huge, barrack-like buildings, housing in over-crowded and very formal conditions too large numbers of multiply handicapped patients who live out over-structured, encapsulated lives away from their fellow citizens. The point should be made, however, that it is only perhaps in the past 20 years that both professionals and lay people have thought of any type of hospital as being other than an organic part of a unified active community. Hunter (1973), in an interesting comment on changing patterns of organisation and management in hospitals for the handicapped, writes:

> If it is important to alter our perspective from one which sees the mentally handicapped primarily in stigmatising or pathological terms to one which emphasizes their 'walking' rather than their 'limping', this does not mean that the essential *pathos* of their situation (Matza, 1969) can be dissipated in facile (and subtly coercive) philosophies of normalisation, which too easily discount, not only clinical but also social and political realities, e.g. higher survival rates among the most severely subnormal and the aged (Cunningham, 1971) and the increasing rationality of modern society which may make it very difficult for the mentally handicapped to find employment.

Hunter is critical of extreme groups who would plead for the total discarding of hospitalisation beyond those needs experienced by normal members of society. He feels that this is pushing logic too far and goes on:

> To plead for the abandonment of Victorian type hospital provision for the mentally handicapped is one thing—to throw specialised hospital provision, as such, out of the window altogether is quite another; and to polarise the situation for the mentally handicapped by creating an artificial dichotomy between the hospital and the community is a way of *not* seeing the real problem, which is how to restore the hospital to the community and the community to the hospital *and how to transform them both in doing so.*
> ... Transformed, normalised, properly sited and, above all, outward

looking hospitals, linked to other hospitals, will continue to be necessary, as will professional teaching and research. One of the objectives for the future must be the creation of reasonably small, de-institutionalised settings for the mentally handicapped, which will act as 'slowed down' centres of excellence, and as agencies for creating and diffusing throughout the larger society, new insights and new values.

If then it seems likely that psychologists and others will live with institutions of one sort or another, hopefully becoming better integrated in the wider community, psychologists will have to exercise both administrative and social psychological skills in maintaining the dynamic bonds between the institution and society as a whole. They will necessarily become preoccupied too with the social structure and nature of the internal organisation in which they work, just as will their colleagues working as community, educational and occupational psychologists have to be apprised of the special pressures and conditions that operate in more formal institutional settings upon the services on which they will from time to time have to call.

The Total Institution and the Medical Model

Although the *Concise Oxford Dictionary* defines an 'institution' as 'an organisation for the promotion of some public object, or the building used by this', this is an over-simplification, necessitating that it be clearly distinguished from what Goffman (1961) has defined as 'the total institution'. Goffman, very early in his illuminating and provocative essay on this topic, points out how among all the institutions available to us in Western society there are some which tend to enclose and restrict people in a way which is very much more extreme than other institutions do. Indeed he points out how they can be rank ordered in terms of this variable of restrictiveness. The latter is often pointed up and symbolised by such characteristics as physically high walls, spaces between the institution and other buildings, barbed wire, locked doors and other features of the structure which have the effect of limiting social interaction with the outside world and imposing other limitations on ingress and egress to and from the institution. As institutions become more shut in from the rest of the environment such movement is difficult to negotiate or to achieve.

The 'total institution' has been described by Goffman as 'a place of residence and work where a large number of like-situated individuals cut off from the wider society for an appreciable period of time, together lead an enclosed formally administered brand of life'. He goes on, 'A basic social arrangement in modern society is that the individual tends to sleep, play and work in different places, with different coparticipants, under different authorities and without an overall rational plan'. In a total institution, however, it is clear that life is just the opposite of this. In fact what happens is that each phase of a patient's daily activity tends to be carried out with many others around him, all of whom are doing the same thing, are being treated more or less alike and are performing as it were, by numbers. Only in a very few instances does this occur in normal life. All phases of the day's activities in a total institution (or sometimes the lack of these) tend to be tightly scheduled and programmed beforehand by a set of rules or explicit formal orders originating from a body of officials or professionals. While this might be the ordinary person's lot for nearly 8 hours of his day, it is certainly not the case for 24 hours of his day.

A further important characteristic of the total institution is that there tends to be a significant and fairly fundamental dichotomy between the large, managed and manipulated group which we like to call patients or residents, and what is generally a relatively smaller number of supervisory or therapeutic staff. This difference is emphasized by the fact that the former tend to have very restricted contact with the outside world whereas the latter often operate on a shift system and are quite well integrated socially into the world around them, moving much more freely in and out of the ward and the community. Patients often say: 'Yes, but you can come and go any time you like!' One needs only to 'shadow' a given patient for the course of a day to see how very restricted their ambit of movement is. The third characteristic is, of course, that social mobility between the two strata of patients and staff tends to be restricted. This is an entirely superimposed reduction of social mobility and one can often see how it is maintained by the organisational difficulties that seem to accrue when, for example, an ex-member of staff has to be admitted to something like a mental deficiency hospital or psychiatric hospital following an acute psychosis or a brain damaging trauma. The more senior the individual was in the hierarchy of the institution the more difficult becomes the adaptation to the new roles that are appropriate to everyone concerned. We may note also how quickly the titles of Mr, Mrs or Miss are omitted from patients' names especially in long stay hospitals but by contrast how staff cling to titles such as Nurse, Sister or Nursing Officer. One result of this is that the nature of communication between these two strata tends to be limited and formalised so that a great deal of information about decisions made about the patients tends to be unknown to the latter and may be distorted in its journey down through the hierarchy of the staff.

The charactetistically fairly wide social gulf between staff and patients in a total institution is generally maintained by the imposition of a fairly systematic system of rulings commonly associated with a number of clearly defined rewards or privileges held out in exchange for conformity to staff established mores. Patient activity tends consequently to be geared very much to acceptance of these imposed rules and privileges. Goffman (1961) comments that there are some special features of the privilege system which should be noted. First, punishments and privileges are themselves modes of organisation peculiar to total institutions. Whatever their severity, punishments are largely known in the inmate's home world as something applied to animals and children; 'this conditioning, behaviouristic model is not widely applied to adults, since failure to maintain required standards typically leads to indirect disadvantageous consequences and not the specific immediate punishment at all. And privileges in the total institution, it should be emphasised, are not the same as perquisites, indulgences, or values, but merely the absence of deprivations one ordinarily expects to have to sustain. The very notions of punishments and privileges are not ones that are cut from civilian cloth'.

Second, the question of release from the total institution is elaborated into the privilege system. Some acts become known as ones that mean an increase or no increase in length of stay, while others become known as means for shortening the sentence.

Third, punishments and privileges come to be geared into a residential work system. Places of work and places to sleep become clearly defined as places where certain kinds and levels of privileges are obtained, and inmates are shifted very frequently and visibly from one place to another as the administrative device for giving them the punishment or reward their co-operativeness warrants. 'The inmates are moved, the system is not' (p. 51).

Later in his essay, Goffman goes on to suggest that there is a mutual incompatibility between total institutions and the family unit. Indeed he points out that the possibility of recourse to the family on the part of the staff in the total institutions is one of the intensifying features of the cleavage between staff and patients in such institutions. There is also support in his contention for smaller ward units and 'family' structure within units in our existing institutions. He goes on, 'Whether a particular total institution acts as a good or a bad force in civil society, force it will have, and this will in part depend on the suppression of a whole circle of actual or potential households. Conversely, the formation of households provides a structural guarantee that total institutions will not be without resistance. Incompatibility of these two forms of social organisation should tell us something about the wider social function of them both'. He goes on, 'The total institution is a social hybrid, part residential community, part formal organisation; therein lies its special sociological interest. There are other reasons for being interested in these establishments too. In our society, they are the forcing houses for changing persons; each is a natural experiment on what can be done to the self'. A primary function of the psychologist is therefore to break down as many of the characteristics of the total institution as possible. Barriers between staff, staff and patients and between all these and the community must be removed, or at least, lowered.

Institutions, like psychologists, vary in size, age, function and efficiency. They have, however, in common certain notable characteristics so deeply inherent in them that those psychologists who work in them may, in spite of a cultivated capacity for detachment and analysis, require a Goffman or some similar critic from outside the institution to remind us of them. Other clinicians may even prefer the uncomplicated encapsulation within a rigidly defined system with limited communication links and executive scope, partly because they are landed with it willy-nilly or partly because they may feel it arrogant to do otherwise. Since the early and skilful outline by Stanton & Schwartz (1954) of the problems of the 'underlife' of the institution and the more recent work by Wing (1962) on institutionalisation of psychotic patients there have been only a few careful studies of these social processes, one or two narrative descriptions such as that by by Russell Barton (1961), but generally a good deal of interest on the part of many psychologists in what can be done to minimise the progression from institution to total institution of many hospitals and units in which clinical psychologists operate. Caudill, Redlick, Gilmore & Brody (1952) have looked at the social structure in single psychiatric wards and Sutherland, Butler, Gibson & Graham (1954) have made a further socio-metric analysis of institutionalised defectives but until more recent publications on the general process of normalisation, usually in relation to subnormality hospitals, by Zarfas (1970), Gunzburg (1970) and by Clark (1968) there had been a dearth of literature making an explicit attempt to deal with these topics.

Many psychologists are unhappily aware of how closely the institutions in which they work, especially geriatric and mental subnormality hospitals, may resemble such a total institution and recognise also the importance of modifying the state of affairs so that in Gunzburg's (1970) words the institution rather 'offers full preparation for normal life to those who can benefit' without 'giving up the role as a protective corner within the normal community. ... If the institution is to provide experience to further the aims of habilitation it follows that its climate, environment, the rhythm of living and the occupation and leisure activities should be as near life (outside) as possible to be preparatory to the stage of comparatively independent life in the open community and to counteract the faulty and inadequate experience of the past'.

The clinical psychologist, being the person in an institution who is most committed to analysis of what is going on in that institution as an organisation is the person who, by training and attitude as well as by virtue of being a participant observer, is best equipped to mediate the process of change. Horsley (1962) has commented on the importance of the therapeutic climate of staff relationships in a subnormality unit and Clark (1970) has, in this connection, further argued that one of the key reasons for the psychologist being the most likely person to involve himself in such issues is that both the nature and manipulation of interpersonal relationships in large hospitals, and especially in mental subnormality hospitals, are constrained by two factors; the characteristics of the hospital as a total institution, and secondly, the fact that the organisational structure and ethos of such hospitals has tended in the past to follow the medical model—a model which is not entirely appropriate to the aims and activities of such a hospital where several different types of personnel may be attempting to carry out several different sorts of task with several different sorts of subject.

The long history of medicine has been one in which people with some malfunction of bodily processes have turned to the doctor who has given them his professional services in a professional and technical relationship in order to remedy the disorder at the patient's request. Even in medieval times the 'casting out of devils' came to be seen as less the concern of the priest and more of the doctor. So madness was not badness and became illness. However, psychiatry, born thus, has over the years been presented with more and more tasks which tend to be out of the compass of traditional medical skills as they were founded in the biological sciences and applied through the hierarchical system of doctor, clinical clerk, matron, sister and nurse, with the patient at the foot rather than at the top of this hierarchy (with the possible exception of private patients). The more authoritarian and God-like the psychiatrist, the more likely he is to pronounce on areas of knowledge and expertise outwith his specific competence and only the more aware and advanced contemporary psychiatrists like J D Haldane (1972) can comment that, 'Because of the lingering respect for medical authority so important in matters of life and death, there is frequently an over eager readiness to seek a psychiatrist's opinion or accept his "prescription" e.g., to transfer a child from one school to another, commit him for Approved School training or remove him from the care of his parents. Psychiatrists have to be careful not to use their *medical* authority in "any activity in which disciplined medical procedures have no part" especially in those cases which can be described as "medical" only by distorting their nature or denying some of their components'.

If an institution's life is dominated by purely medical considerations then the tendency will indeed be for the patient to be at the foot of the power-structure rather than at the top. This is seen with most emphasis in the general hospital. In the words of Gerda Cohen (1964) 'although the hospital operates ostensibly for patients alone (not to provide jobs or help a consultant with his career) their status is low; level with the ward maid or perhaps an assistant porter. The chain of command goes from top to bottom; from matron and senior medical staff down through each grade to the junior nurse. Information on what is happening at the bottom percolates with difficulty through to the top. The bigger the hospital the more attenuated the lines of communication and the stronger the tendency to work in water-tight compartments with only formal contact between each. Thus we find most rigid hierarchies in hospitals of over a thousand beds where staff cannot possibly know each other. Psychiatric hospitals are crippled by their size, like a dinosaur whose nervous system has not kept up with evolution'.

When a patient enters a mental subnormality, and very often a psychiatric, hospital the situation is not, in fact, analogous to a patient entering a general hospital for an appendectomy or control of renal infection where there is a clear-cut relation of server and served between doctor and patient. Rather does one find this relationship one of governor and governed. As soon as this happens the whole frame of reference against which a patient's behaviour is judged undergoes a translation from the terms in which it would be observed and modified in life outside to medical terms. As Goffman (1961) has it, 'interpersonal happenings are transferred into the patient, establishing him as a relatively closed system that can be thought of as pathological and correctable. Thus, if a patient tends to argue vigorously with the charge nurse on how he spends his patient allowances or pocket money this is seen not as an exercise of his individual autonomy but as an example of irritability and aggressiveness and goes down in the case notes in the latter terms. Similarly, when patients in group therapy make complaints about conditions or staff behaviour to a psychotherapist there is a tendency for the latter to suggest that the patient deal with this by re-arranging his own internal world and not by the therapist's attempting to alter activities or organisation of the other agents. Moreover, as O'Hara (1968) a nurse himself, has pointed out, a nurse's training not only inculcates in him the view of the patient as 'suffering from an illness' rather than having difficulties with certain life situations but also fashions the manner as well as the content of the thinking. Nursing, until very recently, has tended to depend on near servility to medical staff but to few others and very seldom to patients. Nursing depends on established procedures: in a given situation you do this or that. One is 'cushioned with routine but the price paid is rigidity of thought'. The ward is not a home but a clinical setting. Hygiene takes precedence over homeliness. In this setting relationships between staff and patients are bound to be formal, if not hostile. Gunzburg & Gunzburg (1970) have indeed illustrated how the nurse's traditional role in mental deficiency of 'supervising storing arrangements', dispensing medicines and administering to ensure food and clothing for patients has waned in favour of her role as a social educator which she has not so far seen as an integral part of her role, nor has has she been specifically trained for it nor given equipment and facilities to carry it out.

The Clinical Psychologist's Role

While it was possible for Gunzburg (1956) in the original paper on the role of the clinical psychologist in a mental subnormality hospital to declare that 'the psychologist as a member of the clinical team of a mental deficiency hospital is a fairly recent innovation and his contribution to clinical work is still barely defined' this is no longer a tenable position. The merest glance at the literature, not only at the vast diversity of single papers but also at the numerous basic texts such as those by the Clarkes (1974) and by Mittler (1970) leaves one in little doubt that the position is much more as reviewed by Clark (1968, 1970). The increasing interest of the Departments of Education and Science and of Social Services in the hospital scene, particularly with regard to mental subnormality, has also not only reduced the professional isolation of psychologists in subnormality hospitals but has also broken down tendencies to total institutionalisation and a preoccupation with the medical model of the hospital as a social organisation. These influences are bound to increase the development of a multidisciplinary approach to the problem presented by subnormality and by institutions themselves and to focus interest on developmental and psychological aspects rather than on the biological, genetic or purely medical issues. It is not intended that these issues should in any way be minimised and there are areas where the greatest of contributions can be made by physicians and geneticists to the welfare of individual patients. It is rather a difference of emphasis so that the on-going social and personal life and welfare of large numbers of patients are being looked at by personnel informed more by the body of clinical and social psychological knowledge rather than by the eye of the physician informed by general medicine and a special expertise in the curing of illness and disease.

The particular role which a given psychologist will play in his institution tends to be determined by his professional experience in other institutions (and to some extent his seniority will reflect this), by his personal qualities and temperament, and not least by the nature of his appointment as described in terms of his contract. Regardless of the latter, there can be little doubt that when a psychologist has formed a certain view of himself his whole style of behaviour will reflect this, his ego identity will be sustained by his ongoing behaviour and he will tend to react fairly sharply if others do not adopt the appropriate behaviour towards him. In view of this, he may bring with him a credit or debit balance to his new appointment depending on the nature of the ego identity that has been built up by his past experience at university, in hospital and elsewhere. The psychologist who comes to a new post as a Principal or Consultant grade psychologist is going to have a much more strongly formulated and substantially based sense of his role than will someone who has just graduated from the probationary grade and is entering his first main institution as a single handed psychologist. Indeed it is not unlikely that these situational factors will be overweening and will crowd out personality differences which might either boost or detract from the personal contribution of that psychologist.

There are, of course, powerful formative infuences brought to bear on the psychologist before he enters an institution at all. Argyle (1964) in asking himself apropos of role behaviour 'what makes the behaviour, attitudes and personality of foremen different from those of psychologists, monks, all-in wrestlers or undertakers' points out that it is due first of all to selection—both self-selection by those who are attracted towards particular positions, and selection by the organisation which employs them. In the second place, role behaviour is the result of carefully designed training courses and of spontaneously created initiation ceremonies. Thirdly, new members are exposed to the actual demands of the job, as well as social pressures to perform it in a certain way.

If the psychologist is to function effectively in an institution in the role adumbrated here, there are certain practicalities which cannot be disregarded. These are that he tends to take up an appointment loaded with appropriate sapiential authority but with very little structural or line authority vis a vis any other professional except the more junior ones in his own department. Nursing, medical and administrative structures do have fairly clear lines of management authority running down through the hierarchy in each case. There is, however, a good deal of debate about inter-relationships between such hierarchies and although a great deal of lip service is paid to 'multidisciplinary efforts' there are sometimes real hazards in seeing this work properly which derive from this lack of a clear awareness of how sapiential and structural authority should interact. One point at which the psychologist can intervene actively to achieve some kind of formal structure of the role he will play is in discussing and finally formulating his contract of employment with the Health Board which employs him. There is a strong case for ensuring that the bare contract of employment in the form of a letter or contract which meets all the necessary statutory and Whitley Council requirements should be modified so that there is some amplification and specification in areas of competence, responsibility and executive authority. This is often done by developing a job description which will be agreed by the clinical psychologist's peer group and co-professionals alike. This may be quite a difficult job description to draw up when an employing authority is not used to appointing psychologists and where it is not in a position to take advice from sufficiently senior people in the profession employed by cognate authorities. Naturally it is frequently to the psychologist's advantage to collaborate with the administrative, medical and other staff who will be concerned with his later functioning in the hospital service and to have both informal and formal discussions about the content of his contract before it is finally mutually agreed. Clearly such a contract should carry a clause allowing for variation at some future time by mutual agreement.

Most social psychologists see the matter of social organisation versus individual needs as something depending on the relative needs for power and for affiliation expressed by individuals within the organisation. Indeed, it is the resolution of this conflict that compelled Brown (1954) and Karlsen (1951) to recognise that social organisations rarely function quite as the organisation chart on the wall would lead one to expect with its nice clear-cut lines of authority and communication, its simply hierarchical ramifications and neat little boxes of responsibility. For a variety of reasons people who should work together may find it difficult to do so and easier to establish working relationships with those to whom they have no formal links within the structure of the organisation. Essentially it can be said that the degree of satisfaction experienced by members of an organisation depends on the congruence between structure and individual needs (Argyle, 1964). Argyris (1957) and others have even considered that there is a basic incongruity between the needs of a mature personality and the requirements of industrial organisations, and they stress the fact that one need which is often not satisfied by the formal structure of organisations is the need for affiliation, with business and professional contacts tending to be cold and often impersonal or alternatively restrained and unspontaneous so as not to disturb the even tenor of the ways of one's colleagues.

Personal Social Skills

Into this organisational jungle can be thrust the fresh young clinical psychologist wielding with delight his highly reliable though sometimes limited cognitive tests and assuring himself of both band-width and fidelity by clutching in one clammy paw a TAT and in the other an EPI. Not only may he hold a Master's degree but he may also be well endowed with 'accurate empathy, non-possessive warmth and genuineness'. He may well find that the institutional world is his oyster but that he requires to assume more than the simple professional role defined by his university course if he is to crack the outer shell and seek the inner pearl. This writer's thesis is that he requires at least two other subroles, that of the organisational executive and that of the deliberate social engineer; and further, not all personalities are likely to be equally equipped to assume these roles.

Now it is clear that degrees, even post graduate degrees in clinical psychology do not in themselves confer on the holder a particular skill in social organisation or in personal relationships but it is well known that there are some people who are good at particular social skills, like interviewing, psychotherapy, persuasion, teaching or selling. What is not known is how general such skills are; whether a person who is good at one of these is also good at the others, whether being good he knows he is good, or being bad, he knows he is bad at these. However, there is some evidence that such skills can be acquired in a way analogous to the learning of motor skills, such as by watching an expert practitioner and by trying out techniques with some feedback on one's performance being available very much as one would learn to play golf, drive a motor car or do well on the ski slopes. So far as salesmen are concerned, demonstration and role playing will often be considered to be helpful and some social skills can be helped by the exercise of working in T groups and other techniques of group analysis. Argyle (1964) has also pointed out that individuals have a characteristic style of interaction in that they try to elicit the desired responses from other people in characteristic ways which might include the speed and extent of their conversation, the degree of their narcissism or the use of the techniques of humour, whimsicality or flattery. Indeed he points out that it is these characteristic modes of expression which are remembered about people and which are thought of as individualising characteristics. Colleagues may help to pinpoint these skills. Single-handed psychologists are at a disadvantage here, both as learners and as exponents.

Social psychologists have frequently confirmed that if a person is rewarded or reinforced for using some particular technique of social behaviour then he is quite likely to use it more frequently, whereas if he receives negative reinforcement then this behaviour will be stamped out. Krasner (1958) has shown that the frequency of making suggestions in a social situation is very much changed even within a few minutes by techniques of negative reinforcement of an entirely social type even when the subjects who are making the suggestions are quite unaware that this has happened. These negative reinforcements might include a failure to agree with, a failure to look the subject in the eye, or a positive expression of boredom or contempt or disgust. Indeed, one of the writer's associates in the local golf club was cured of what his colleagues described as 'I disease' by this very technique: his habit of saying how 'I scored a birdie at the 7th', 'I played a great shot from the rough at the 17th' etc was negatively reinforced by the physical distance between himself and his listeners being rapidly increased and by the assumption of expressions of glazed vacuity on the part of those compelled to listen. Those of us, however, who are extraverted stable individuals will be particularly interested in the work of Haythorn (1953) which showed that adjusted extraverted people tend to facilitate friendly relationships within groups and an easy-going productive atmosphere, whereas withdrawn, schizoid people produce a tense uneasy atmosphere, and psychopaths may disrupt the group entirely by increasing sources of tension and conflict. In this way it is clear that separate single individuals can largely affect the way of life of a group, contribute to the formation of new groups and change group norms or standards. Further, there will be differences in the ability of individuals to be influential in this way and each to become a well accepted member of the group who wields this influence and makes new suggestions to the mutual advantage of the members. Even when techniques are made available to the layman as by Stephen Potter (1952) these individual differences will still give certain people an advantage in face to face social situations even in the field of vigorous ploys and counter ploys.

The Psychologist's Traditional Professional Role

Most clinical psychologists come to an institution expecting to play the professional role only and this is one for which their previous training has prepared them well. It is easily understood and by many co-professionals thought to be the only role that the psychologist should properly pursue. This is the role in which the psychologist will be concerned inevitably with psychological testing and diagnosis, the on-going assessment of patients, research of both an *ad hoc* or fundamental kind, counselling, psychotherapy or behaviour therapy, the planning of rehabilitation, training and so on. The exercise of this fairly technological function predicates certain basic relationships being established with both patients and colleagues. In the case of the former the psychologist will tend to establish warm, interested and supportive rapport with a large number of patients in the hospital and he will be seen by them as a non-threatening but relatively important figure who seems to move among them and among other staff at all levels with equal ease. Where the psychologist has established a strong therapeutic as distinct from research role his commitment to patients will be seen even more clearly and he will perhaps have stronger identification with them than with the other professional groupings within the hospital. It is also relatively easy for staff to form some stereotyped notion as to what the psychologist's role is when they see him behave in this more or less traditional way. There is, however, a tendency, in nursing staff particularly, to focus largely on the testing aspect of the psychologist's work and perhaps to some degree on his or her research, but nursing staff often have greater difficulty in conceptualising the therapeutic role of the psychologist, whether this is expressed directly in individual psychotherapy and behaviour therapy or more subtly in 'natter groups', case conferences or on ward rounds. In the eyes of many nurses the psychologist is thought of as aligning himself with them so long as he is testing and researching but as tending to align himself with patients and to effect changes which might on occasions undermine the authority of the nurse when he is functioning as a therapist or counsellor. This can promote some anxiety that he may not be aligned with the institutional mores supported by the medical model, and the nurses often become more apprehensive about what goes on behind closed doors when the psychologist has a counselling session than by what goes on behind the same doors when he is applying test techniques. Good working relationships, therefore, depend on their getting adequate and prompt feedback about this in terms that they can understand.

The Executive Role of the Psychologist

The executive role of the psychologist is taken to include those tasks where he is exercising control over the disposal of patients to rehabilitation and training procedures, very often in association with therapeutic measures resulting from counselling or behaviour therapy; those where he has line management responsibility for staff/patient relationships; and those where he is explicitly concerned with the efficiency or development of communication lines including effective feedback mechanisms (Clark, 1970). In the post-Trethowan era many heads of psychology departments and even heads of sub-sections of the department such as units concerning themselves with the clinical sub-specialities of mental handicap, geriatrics and child or adolescent psychology will have management or executive responsibilities. These will be concerned with the deployment of staff, the logistics of running a sub-department in a district or hospital and of organising workflow, team research and so forth.

In subnormality and psychiatric hospitals in particular, many members of staff in the non-medical, non-nursing substructure of the hospital who are quite unaware of the psychologist's professional role, see him only in his executive function. This generates relatively little conflict because the gardener, plumber or laundry manager are interested much more in what information the psychologist can give about helping to deal with patients than about how this information was generated. Not only that, but they tend to locate the psychologist more in the clinical hierarchy than in their own staff structure and, therefore, communication between himself and them is across hierarchies rather than up and down one pyramidal structure of authority. In this executive role he is often difficult to locate for other members of staff because he is continually breaking down the boundary between sub-groups and the pattern of institutional mores. He will often, for example, be equally as concerned about behaviour and attitudes of staff as about the behaviour and attitudes of patients. He will be as concerned about the relationships established between, say, the assistant psychiatrist and the patient and himself, as about the relationship between a plumber and that patient or between an occupational therapist and some senior nurses and so on. He therefore has to assume a roving commission across the pyramids of the different power structures within the hospital and many of the difficulties of relationships at the executive level are generated by the fact that on the one hand he is trying to break down long established hierarchies among staff and on the other trying to diminish any of the boundaries between staff and patient which institutions tend to elaborate and emphasize (Goffman, 1961).

The traditional tripartite organisation of many hospitals defines at least three main authority hierarchies; the first, comprising psychiatric, medical and psychological and other professional personnel, the second being the nursing structure and the third being the authority of the administrator or hospital secretary. However, in a subnormality hospital, the psychologist may find himself in a situation whereby, for example, he must involve all of those structural units when he wishes to transfer a patient from general nursing care and occupational therapy on the ward into a work unit under an industrial supervisor or into one of the artisan sections of the hospital, and also to change the patient's pocket money and parole arrangements in line with prevailing incentive schemes. This necessitates initiating nursing staff action, modifying administrative procedures and correlating this with the medical requirements of the case so that here again the psychologist has to intervene in the three different pyramids without in fact disturbing the stability of any of these. It is not difficult to achieve this when all the members in the different hierarchies are agreed about the disposal of the patient; but if it means, for example, that the ward is to be deprived of an efficient ward worker, who has relieved the nursing staff of rather tedious duties, or if it means that extra clerical work is to be carried by some of the secretarial staff in order for revised rates of pay to be granted, then quite sophisticated techniques of interpersonal manipulation based on an on-going trustful and relaxed relationship will become necessary.

When he is functioning in his clinical role as a professional or even to some extent as an organisational executive the clinical psychologist will be exercising what is frequently described as sapiential authority, as distinct from structural authority which is exercised by virtue of a stated formal position in a power structure laid down either by contract or by other published documents. The distinction between these two kinds of authority is well made in Appendix 1, page 117, of the Salmon Report on the organisation of the Nursing Profession. *Structural authority* is defined as 'the right, vested in the position and so the role of manager, to command and to expect and enforce obedience of others in order that the function of managing (advising and coordinating) may be fulfilled. The right stems from the necessity for management. (It is sometimes called *line authority*)'. By contrast, *sapiential authority* is 'the right, vested in a person, to be heard by reason of expertness of knowledge—just as one person, relative to another, may be an "authority" on a particular subject. (It is sometimes referred to as *staff authority* and does not involve structural authority, the right to command).' 'Structural authority, which stems from the position a manager assumes, is enhanced by his personal, sapiential authority, recognised in promotion by merit ... A person who exercises sapiential authority advises, instructs (meaning teaches) and informs and is said to *direct* others (as distinct from control, implying command). A person directed is not obliged to act upon the advice, instruction or information of the one who directs, as distinct from being obliged to obey the rightful order of one who controls'. It is later added, of course, that coordination of functions can be carried out by the exercise either of structural or sapiential authority, that is, by control or direction.

Another way of looking at this contrast of authorities is to suggest that, in the informal organisation of the institution, sapiential authority will be more heavily weighted whereas in the formal organisation of the institution structural authority will carry more weight. The latter is certainly more important where issues described above arise, in that the clinical psychologist has to initiate activities involving the disposal of patients and others which can only be fulfilled by the intermediacy of other professions each of which is often itself independent and may have a very clearcut and sometimes tightly defined structural authority as, for example, in nursing where, since the Salmon Report, job evaluations for particular grades are very specifically laid down.

This situation may be complicated even more for particular professions within the structure where these professions like medicine and clinical psychology have not only their own hierarchies of sapiential and structural authority within departments as, for example, where the consultant looks after his team of senior registrars, registrars, HSOs and housemen and the Area Psychologist will be responsible for principal psychologists, senior psychologists, basic grades and post graduate students etc, but each has also an advisory structure which may be an effective channel of communication between the body of the profession and the employers of these professionals such as Health Boards. Such advisory groups will have their own often elected chairman who may not always coincide with the appointed heads of department and there is therefore room for conflict where the advice given to the employer by the head of department does not appear to be immediately congruent with that given by the advisory groups. It is on these occasions that the informal structure of the organisation is most likely to have its own peculiar potency.

The Psychologist as a Social Engineer

The third role of the clinical psychologist, as a social engineer, has not in the past been given much attention by clinical psychologists generally, partly because it has heretofore been seen as outside his brief and partly because his postgraduate training has biased him to tread only the somewhat surer ground of what has been described above as his professional role. Nevertheless, even an acquaintanceship with social psychology based only on his undergraduate training is sufficient to show how its general principles lend themselves to being exercised within the context of institutions. There are in fact relatively few other people in the hosital staff structure who have the same opportunities to move freely amongst all personnel in the hospital and indeed it is one of the worst characteristics of total institutions that personnel in different specialties can so easily become encapsulated into their own departments, the stereotypes of their attitudes and behaviour becoming in consequence more rigid.

Social psychology has generated a wide variety of experimental results which can be summarised and presented in a way indicating the very potent position of the clinical psychologist in an institution to modify behaviour and attitudes according to principles which are clearly agreed with immediate professional colleagues and, if necessary, the employing authority. An ethical difficulty arises, however, in that the clinical psychologist can use these same techniques to persuade both of the latter that his methods are not only defensible but desirable and, as Smail (1970) has pointed out, this is a heavy responsibility to bear. Perhaps one of the advantages of a rather cumbersome democracy is the process of dilution which is undergone by attempts to change attitudes and behaviour through the process of committees, commissions and the decisions of individual officers following these.

It may be useful at this point to review in outline form some of the findings which relate different variables to attitude change. It is worth remembering, as Zimbardo & Ebbeson (1969) point out, that all techniques of attitude change rely on the assumption that change comes out of conflict, discrepancy, inconsistency or discontent with the status quo. It is not enough simply for the social engineer to propagate a generalised atmosphere of sweetness and light. His business will, on the contrary, often be that of introducing elements of conflict in a controlled manner and later of introducing solutions which may reduce this—a process of constructive dissonance, so to speak. None recognised this better than Nicolo Machiavelli (1469–1527): 'It must be considered that there is nothing more difficult to carry out, more doubtful of success, no more dangerous to handle, than to initiate a new order of things; for the reformer has enemies in all those who profit by the old order, and only lukewarm defenders in all those who would profit by the new order, this lukewarmness arising partly from the credulity of mankind, who do not truly believe in anything new until they have had actual experience of it'.

Morris (1969, 1972) clearly recognises this relationship between conflict between and within organisations and different forms of structure. Essentially she sees the conflict as being about power, status, and the use of scarce resources. If there is no competitive conflict about these, people are complacent with the status quo and there is no change. The structure of an organisation such as the NHS, for example, she sees as being complicated by the overlapping concerns of the three main hierarchies, medicine, nursing and the administration, and conflict here can be resolved only by an effective communication system, both formal and informal, which flows both vertically and horizontally.

As a social engineer, the psychologist within an institution is likely to be much concerned with communications and with producing attitude change in both staff and patients. This may often be a more taxing task than it might seem, depending on the size of institution, because of the uncertainty created by the distinctions betwen sapiential and line management authority. Nevertheless, Zimbardo & Ebbesen (1969) have suggested that one descriptive schema for categorising the many known variables in attitude change which such a psychologist might constantly bear in mind is contained by the simple sentence: 'Who says what, to whom, and with what effect?'. This phrase allows one to organise one's knowledge of social psychology under the headings of the communicator or source of information; the message conveyed; the audience or recipients of that message, and finally, of the dimensions of the response to it. It could be added that one should be concerned also with two items not included in the paradigm, the medium of transmission of the message and the situation in which the message is received.

The following summary of social psychological findings which bear on this function of the psychologist is borrowed largely from Zimbardo & Ebbesen (1969) who have collated most relevant findings from social psychology. They concern themselves with (a) *the persuader,* then with (b) *how to present the issues,* followed by the consideration of (c) *the audience* as a group of individuals, (d) *the influence of groups* and finally (e) with the *persistence* of opinion change.

Dealing first with the characteristics of the persuader, they indicate that there will tend to be an opinion change in the desired direction both if the communicator has characteristics which show him to be easily believed rather than of low credibility. The two factors which are likely to promote high credibility are a demonstrably high level of expertise with a wide knowledge of the issues presented and, secondly, an appearance to those concerned of trustworthiness and of having an appropriate motivation to present knowledge in a reasonably unbiased way. It should be noted nevertheless that the credibility of the persuader in this sense plays a much smaller part later on as information is assimilated than it does immediately after the subject is exposed to the material for the first time. At the time of the immediate exposure, communicator characteristics irrelevant to the topic of his message such as mannerisms, bizarre or unconventional ways of dress and so forth, may influence favourably or otherwise the acceptance of the message. The psychologist may therefore have to depend on his colleagues to give him insight into such idiosyncratic characteristics as might unfavourably influence such an impact. It is also known that the effectiveness of a particular persuader is increased if he starts off by expressing views consistent with some of those held by his listeners even if he intends to deviate from these later in the presentation. There is also a reciprocal quality between what the audience thinks of a persuader and of his message so that if they think highly of him they will think highly of the message and if they think highly of this message they may take the view that the persuader is himself someone of value. Social psychology has also demonstrated empirically, as has the evidence of trade union and other negotiation, that the more extreme the opinion change the communicator asks for the more actual change he is likely to get. This, however, is true only up to a certain limit since with extreme discrepancy between the two and, in particular, when sources of attitude change have low credibility then the resulting change will be much less marked.

It will be clear therefore that if the psychologist is going to be an effective persuader he cannot expect change to be over-rapid or dramatic. In the first place if he is to gain the credibility he requires he has to have time to demonstrate his expertise and his knowledge of the issues at stake. However, that knowledge must be well-founded and must be seen to have been accumulated in a relevant way. If this is not so then he is likely to suffer from the phenomenon of being seen as a new broom who will attempt to sweep clean and will generate the appropriate resistances. If, by contrast, he takes time to operate sensibly, consistently and with an awareness of the specific conditions which he is going to operate in, then his credibility is likely to be increased. Such time is in most institutions likely to be months rather than weeks and possibly even years rather than months. So far as effecting change by making a very substantial demand is concerned, then there can be a critical judgement as to what might be accepted as the highest level demand. For example, if a psychologist were to be anxious to introduce, say, mixed nursing into two wards in a 20 ward hospital, then perhaps it might be wise to ask for consideration of such a scheme in 4 or 5 wards but not in all of them. His negotiating position is then not outrageous but can be pared down to a level which may not be inconsistent with the initial intention.

So far as presentation of the issues is concerned, the first thing to be guarded against is giving cues which forewarn the audience of the attempt to manipulate them by the communication process. Should they sense this, resistance to change is likely and such sensing may be diminished by presenting distractors simultaneously with the message in a way which will decrease resistance to the message. In general, it is advocated that one side of the argument be presented only when the audience is, on the whole, friendly or when the communicator's position is the only one to be presented to them or when immediate change is required even if it needs only to be temporary. However, should the audience begin by disagreeing with the communicator then it is important that both sides of the argument are put, especially when it is highly likely that the audience will hear the other sides of the communicator's argument from individuals outside the present situation. It must be borne in mind that where opposite views are presented one after the other, whether by the same person or by others, the one presented last is the one likely to be effective.

Depending on the type of audience available to the persuader, emotional appeals may be more influential than factual or vice versa. In particular, there will be a greater probability of opinion change in the hoped for direction if the persuader explicitly states conclusions than if the audience is allowed to draw their own, except where the latter is a fairly intelligent one—in which circumstances, implicit conclusion drawing tends to effect nore favourable attitude change. It has also been noted that there is generally a positive relationship between the intensity of fear arousal by the persuader and the amount of change especially if the persuader makes recommendations for action which are both explicit and possible to carry out. If, however, he generates fear and does not make such proposals then the reaction will tend to be negative.

These techniques are most likely to be productive for the psychologist when he is operating in a case conference or administrative meeting type of setting. Some of the distractors mentioned in the paragraphs above may take the form of not so much the cognitive content of what is being said as variations in emotional tone and the interspersing of substantial material for discussion with banter, light conversation, gestures and so forth. In view of the importance of having the last word in a disputative situation this may sometimes be developed by offering a summary of the argument and discussion that has gone before, making sure that the communicator's point of view in the issue is the one which is given last. The extent to which fear arousal might be appropriate in the hospital or institutional setting is perhaps less obvious. There may, however, be times when adverse changes are being imposed when the persuader should suggest that were the information about these changes to get out into the wider world then the press, for example, might be likely to ridicule or lampoon the situation. Thus a mild sort of fear of that kind of unfavourable exposure would be generated to be minimised later by the persuader suggesting a feasible modification of the originally proposed idea.

Turning now to the audience as individuals, it has been noted by many researchers that the people most wanted in an audience by a persuader with a job to do are often the least likely to be present, since natural processes of selectively seeking out information which fits one's personal views are well known. Preaching to the converted achieves little change. Curiously, there is not the same selective avoidance of information which is not consonant with one's current attitude. It is also common sense as well as a phenomenon endorsed by social psychological experimentation that the level of intelligence of an audience will determine the effectiveness of some kinds of appeals and that if persuasion is going to be effective then the reasons underlying attitudes expressed by an audience as well as the attitudes themselves must be tackled by the persuader. Furthermore, audiences may contain a number of individuals who are, in general, more easily persuaded than others, and some whose temporary susceptibility to persuasion will be increased by any circumstances which tend to reduce their self-esteem. By the same token, individuals who are easily persuaded by one persuader are easily persuaded to opposing views by a conflicting persuader. Both common sense and experimentation demonstrate that if subjects are particularly ego-involved in the consequences of an acceptance of change, then the probability of change is increased, and this is greater when the discrepancy of attitudes between source and audience is greater. Finally, and perhaps importantly for the social engineer, any subject who actively role-plays through a previously unacceptable position will tend to accept this much more readily on subsequent occasions.

It will be apparent from the above and from other experiments that we are all much influenced by groups, our opinions and attitudes tending to cohere to a greater or lesser extent with those of the groups to whom we actually belong and wish to belong. Such is the nature of our society that we tend to be rewarded for conforming in this way and to be dealt with harshly when we attempt to deviate from group-accepted norms. The more we tend to cohere with the group the less influenced we are likely to be by conflicting information. This is especially true if members of the group have tended to make their opinions explicit to others in a public situation, thus making it harder to change them than it would have been had they just been privately adopted. Nevertheless, if there is such resistance to attitude and opinion change then it can be diminished by audience participation, including group discussion and decision making by the group. In context, it is worth noting that even if an individual is supported by only one other member in a minority situation he becomes significantly stronger against the majority vote than he would be standing alone. Indeed it has been noted that a minority of two of this type, if they hold their views very consistently and firmly, can have a significant effect on even large majorities holding opposing views.

Finally, so far as the persistence of opinion change is concerned it is apparent that there is a decrement with the passage of time, but there tends to be more rapid decay of attitude change over time as a result of communication from positive sources than from negative sources. Attitude change will on the whole tend to be more persistent over time if the receiver actively participates in behaviour following from his attitude change or growing from it rather than simply being a passive recipient of information. Simple repetition of a communication will of course prolong its influence but in general more complex or subtle messages will produce slower decay of attitude change than very simple stark messages.

It should not be necessary to illustrate in detail many practical applications by the psychologist, both in his executive and social engineering roles, of these principles other than to comment, for example, that there is total obligation on the psychologist to be professionally skilful and to make his aim explicit. It will be particularly apparent from what is written above that one essential for attitude change is for the psychologist to have an audience whether this be a group of patients, a group of administrators, or doctors of a managment unit. For the psychologist to have access to these it is important therefore that his own competence as a persuader with the individual be highly developed and that, as we have noted above, he notes communicator characteristics in himself which are perhaps irrelevant to the content of his message but which may be supportive or destructive of his position, e.g. mode of dress, fluency, nervous habits, dilatoriness and so on.

With regard to the influence of some of the relevant groups among whom he works it is important for the psychologist accurately to define the operating groups within his institution and note the different contacts which predetermine the kind of groups which will emerge, e.g. a psychiatric registrar attending a psychology department seminar on test construction will be subject to identification pressures within this group which will dissipate as soon as he moves into a purely medical context with his professional equals but the increased expertise he has gained will give him a dominance in the latter group which, if he is going to maintain it, will necessitate a continued affiliation with the former. In the same way, a charge nurse who plays in the same table tennis team for the hospital as the clinical psychologist is going to be more responsive to patient rating techniques suggested by the latter than the nurse who has no such affiliations.

The application of many of these principles would be facilitated by the attendance of the psychologist at as many seminars, coffee room discussions (with as great a multiplicity of staff present as possible), ward meetings, staff group meetings and case conferences as possible, also by a variety of informal relationships such as may be generated in sports or social occasions within the institution.

Communication Links

Consideration of these general principles culled from social psychological writings and applicable by the psychologist in both his executive and social engineering roles leads to a consideration of the existing nature of communication networks in the institution. Once again distinction between the formal and the informal communication network needs to be drawn since the incumbent will very rapidly find that these two do not always coincide. His first task may well be to work out schematically the nature of these network systems on both planes. In a previous paper Clark (1970) has drawn attention to the considerable amount of experimental work on different kinds of communication networks in groups (although not always in hospitals), and some discussion of this is available in Sprott (1958) and Klein (1956).

1. Chain
2. 'Y'
3. Circle
4. Wheel
5. All channel

Types of communication networks

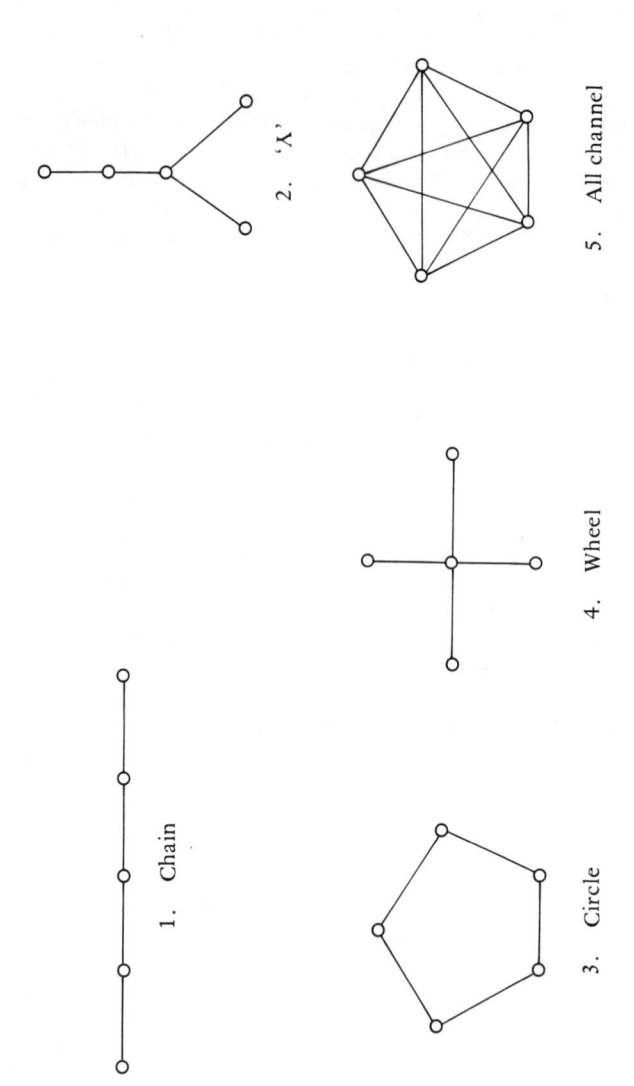

These writers on the basis of both their own work and of earlier studies by Leavitt (1951) concluded that different kinds of communication network tend to be optimal for different purposes. Dubin (1959) suggested that the sheer efficiency of communication could normally be measured in terms of the number of communication links in a given network. The smaller the number of such communication links in a group, the greater will be the efficiency of the group in task performance. There are more links, for example, in the All-channel pattern than in the Circle pattern and more links in the Circle than in the Wheel pattern (see Figure opposite). Efficiency of task performance would therefore be greater in the latter structure. Extending some of Leavitt's (1951) experimental work, Guetzkow & Simon (1955) used five-man groups in which the task was to discover which one of six symbols was held in common by all group members. In the experiment the subjects sat round a circular table with vertical partitions separating them. They were not allowed to talk to one another but communicated by passing messages through slots connecting each position. Each person was given a card with five symbols and on each subject's card the missing symbol was different. Fifty-six groups were randomly assigned by the experimenters to three different networks of communication. In the Circle net, as illustrated, subjects could pass their message to either or both of two neighbours. In the Wheel net there is a key man to whom all four colleagues can communicate and in the All-channel pattern everyone can communicate with everyone else. Since messages have to flow to a decision centre for action and must flow back to the senders to inform them of the decision, the Wheel provides a two level hierarchy and the Circle and All-channel nets a three level hierarchy. In the Circle for example, two neighbours can send information to their opposite neighbours, who in turn relay this information, with their own, to the fifth member. He can then send the solution back to his group, but three levels are involved in the process.

Leavitt (1951) was able to show that the efficiency in speed of problem solving of the Wheel and Y networks were better than the Circle and Chain networks in that the latter used more messages to reach solutions. Yet when errors were made on the Circle network they were more easily corrected than was the case for the other patterns: moreover, the pleasure and satisfaction in participation was found to be greater in the Circle pattern. Guetzkow & Simon (1955) reasoned that the apparent superiority of the two level hierarchy of the Wheel for task accomplishment might simply be due to the time it took for a group to discover and use the optimal organisational pattern for its specific types of net, rather than to the patterns of the networks themselves. They point out that a group assigned to the Circle organisation might spend considerable time in a more complex interaction than the optimal pattern described already. The work later confirmed that when groups in an All-channel or Circle net discovered the optimal organisational pattern they were just as efficient as Wheel groups, for example. They concluded that the advantages for a system which employed fewer links lay not in the efficiency of the simpler network as such, but in the fact that it required little trial and error by the group to use it effectively. Katz & Kahn (1966) have also pointed out that these experiments with the extensiveness and number of links of networks were concerned with task oriented communications. They point out that the conclusions cannot be generalised to socio-emotional or supportive types of communication.

Revans (1964) found a correlation between patterns of communication in hospitals and several indices of efficiency. In hospitals with low wastage of student nurses, slow turnover of senior staff, and rapid discharge of patients, communication between the various groups of people was better than in those with higher student wastage, quicker staff turnover and slower discharge of patients. In the former hospital compared with the latter, the climate was more permissive and less authoritarian; the patients felt more able to question the nurses, student nurses felt they could question the tutors, the sisters the matron, the matron the consultants and so on. There was a general ease of communication both in upwards and downwards directions.

In fact, over-complex communication links are sometimes difficult to cope with for many groups and in later experiments by Guetzkow & Dill (1957) it was found that groups seem to prefer a minimum linkage system. Seventeen out of twenty groups which had started with a pattern permitting ten links had, by the end of 20 trials, cut this to four links. Pressures were generated inside the groups to move towards simpler communication networks and the groups that did not follow such a pattern were less efficient in task accomplishment. One of the common reasons for such organisational structures in communication systems breaking down is that organisations often have communication loops of disproportionate sizes with regard to message sending and message receiving. The top echelon of an organisation can often issue directives, instructions or information for the whole organisation and yet find that this information is stifled at the next level down. The communication system may well involve all levels of organisation on the sending side but only the upper echelon of the receiving side. A system therefore needs to take account of the need for feedback about how far the effects of communication can be observed, quantified and fed back to the original communicator. This is a specially sensitive point where an institution has tended to follow the medical model and where, for example, there may be very adequate communication of a simplified style between consultant, registrar, ward sister and senior nurses, but where in fact there are implications in this communication for a number of other groups, perhaps including psychologists, administrators, and occupational therapists but where, because of the closed loop system of the medical hierarchy, insufficient attention is paid to the need to communicate across sub-systems. The reciprocal breakdown can, of course, also occur. It can be easily seen therefore that there is still a lot of room for further experimental work on such interactions between sub-systems of this sort in institutions and many clinical psychologists will wish to continue assessing and measuring the effects of such communication structures.

It may be interesting to note in passing that not only are there complexities in the communications sub-systems for staff relationships, but that these are found also in interactions among patients and between staff and patients. Miles' (1965) study of some aspects of culture among subnormal hospital patients illustrated the importance of channels of communication between patients and staff and of the need for defined goals and reports of progress. She rightly points out how relatively little is known about the effect of lack of social mobility in such patients and whether this enables them to adjust more easily or whether in fact a rigid hierarchy has an adverse effect on patients' eventual adjustment to outside society. The lack of positive goals that she sees as a disadvantage can, of course, be compensated for by a planned incentive system, and the relative incapacity of individual patients to assess themselves and the attitudes of others to them is similarly something which Clark (1960) has shown can be improved. It is only reasonable that the clinical psychologist in an institution should make a detailed assessment of what is happening in the communication system, and in the needs for power and affiliation that he observes in his colleagues, before attempting to modify any of these. An adoption of the general principle of 'Softly, softly, catches monkey', together with a healthy awareness of the fact that formal and informal organisational systems will coexist, is important for the later effectiveness of the psychologist in his role both as executive and social engineer. Once his preparatory work has been carried out, then it does become possible to see which organisational structures within the institution need to be done away with and which new ones need to be introduced.

Some arrangements which would facilitate the application of many of the principles outlined above include general orientation of the hospital towards a case conference approach to clinical issues, and also the day-to-day running arrangements for the vast majority of patients. It is relevant to note that both the Payne Report on Whittingham Hospital and the Batchelor Report on the Staffing of Subnormality Hospitals in Scotland have come out clearly in favour of a multi-disciplinary approach and a professional executive to control rehabilitation procedures. There is a strong case for regular fixed case conferences together with case conferences which may be called by any member of hospital staff and attended by all who have an interest in the case. Gunzburg (1970) has already indicated that too often the clinical case conference as an attempt to determine an overall strategy to individual problems, appears frequently quite ineffective because it is modelled on medical/psychiatric lines, and may be more concerned with determining the nature of deficiency rather than with investigating the specific action required to ameliorate the consequences of the deficiency. Both Gunzburg and the present writer are agreed that it should be the task of a case conference as it is understood by ourselves to:

(a) take note of a particular training or therapeutic need
(b) decide on a course of action
(c) allocate prime responsibility for initiating action to various disciplines
(d) make everyone concerned aware of the intended action, and
(e) review the effectiveness of the measures taken after a reasonable time interval

It should be noted that though the primary purpose of this arrangement is to initiate definite activity to help a particular patient this will nevertheless assist in triggering off specific changes in practice and outlook throughout the institution which will often be beneficial to many other patients.

Communication systems and the opportunity for attitude change within the staff structure are probably best developed by making arrangements for frequent meetings of both a formal and an informal sort. The latter may well take the form of mixed dining room or an extensive staff room which is essentially multi-disciplinary for all senior staff rather than, for example, having their coffee in separate offices. The development of social club contact and relationships within sports and hobbies between different members of staff can be fostered.

At the more formal level, departmental meetings with periodic inter-departmental meetings should be arranged and although they need not necessarily follow a rigid timetable they should not be allowed to lapse even when long periods of routine seem to suggest that no need for these meetings exists. Ward meetings and seminars with an ostensible teaching function can also be useful opportunities for dissemination of information likely to influence attitudes. And both formal and informal ward rounds by the psychologist, which are entirely open-ended and in which he makes himself available to staff as much as to patients, are similarly valuable. A regional or a hospital newspaper which may be shared as an organ between patients and staff should not be scorned as a medium both for the dissemination of useful information and for the publication of views which may prepare the ground for behavioural and attitude change which is to be more formally initated later.

Patient to patient communication links are already highly organised in most institutions and are frquently semi-illicit: and the more coercive and custodial the regime the more this will be so (Morris, 1972). A diminution of the semi-illicit communications frquently follows on the provision of facilities for a freer inter-communication between patients, and a rich social life will contribute very much to this. Extensive use of a parole system coupled to an incentive scheme together with hospital dances, social club, interward visiting, hobbies, clubs, sports teams and so forth, goes a long way towards this, and the formal training arrangements within the hospital should be similarly geared to the development of social skills, communication skills and co-education. The boundary between group therapy and more general attitude change among patients as a group becomes very ill defined in such a setting.

There are many other specific procedures which the psychologist with an interest in the broader role propounded here will devise for himself in accordance with his particular repertory of social skills and experience. The exercise of structural authority will be most useful to him when he wishes to bring about behavioural changes which will in turn lead to attitude change, but where the reverse is true then his sapiential authority is likely to be most exercised. In fact probably the most effective social engineers are those who have the capacity to bring about change so that those on whom the change is operating either are not aware that it has taken place or think they have initiated it. And the change is likely to be effective where those who have been subject to it endorse either by rationalisation or by conviction the behaviour patterns that have been brought about.

Conclusion

Not all institutions are 'total institutions' and many are now moving away from the medical model of organisation. Some are too large for many of the techniques outlined above to be operable in them as a whole and the first task of the psychologist may be to select out a small sub-section of the institution which can be usefully worked upon and reorganised. There is probably an optimal size of institution for the efficient exercise of these skills, but not enough work appears to have been done to clarify what it may be. Subjective opinion is that it is somewhere around 500 beds but there can be little doubt too that very small institutions of 20–30 beds can still show the influence of both the medical model and of total institutionalisation, so smallness is no guarantee of efficiency and health.

In all institutions there is little doubt that the clinical psychologist has a great deal to contribute in terms of his professional or technical role where he works as a diagnostician on assessment problems, as a rehabilitator and as a therapist with individual and sometimes small groups of patients. His research expertise can apply itself in many fields. Most clinical psychologists in institutions, however, become acutely aware of the undercurrent of tension, disorganisation and conflict that frequently pull them about whether they are fulfilling only a professional role or otherwise, and many clinical psychologists will be aware of how adversely these undercurrents affect the life and welfare of patients. For this reason a strong plea is made for the psychologist to exercise his privileged position and to move towards an adoption of the executive and of the social engineering roles which have been outlined here. The psychologist has the expert awareness of communication systems, interpersonal behaviour, techniques of persuasion and capacity for controlled observation which should equip him first to understand and second to mediate the nature of the organisation within which he operates.

This role imposes considerable ethical pressures on the psychologist which are, as Smail (1970) has pointed out, sometimes inadequately considered.

Indeed, psychologists who have not wholly worked out their ethical position and do not have clear-cut and validated aims and goals which are to emerge from their activity perhaps should not indulge in this role at all. For one thing, the price of making a mistake can be very high not only in terms of the psychologist's own career but in terms of the future life of the institution. Those who grow proud in their power to manipulate events should bear in mind the possibility of a fall and perhaps should also consider a quotation from St Benedict quoted by Cohen (1954) in a totally different context: 'Should there be craftsmen in the monastery, let them exercise their crafts with all humility and reverence, if the Abbot so command. But if one of them grow proud because of the knowledge of his craft, in that he seems to confer some benefit on the monastery, let such a one be taken away from this craft and not practise it again, unless perchance, after he has humbled himself, the Abbot may bid him resume it'.

Abbot Smail's (1970) position is perhaps best represented by a quotation from the recent paper referred to above:

> The most dramatic result of the behaviourist approach in psychology consists in its leading to a view of human relationships which formerly was not widely subscribed to, even by psychologists, but which now threatens to become accepted even outside psychology. To take an example, social psychologists have found it useful to develop objective measures of interpersonal processes such as eye-contact, smiling and so on. From here the step has been taken [unjustifiably in Smail's view] of substituting the technique for the relationship; that is, psychologists have taken these objective indices of psychological events, divorced from their context, and attempted to apply them in social situations in order to 'modify' or 'shape' the behaviour of others. One only can do this if one is willing to discard genuineness as a meaningful concept. Door-to-door salesmen must have anticipated psychologists by decades when it comes to an understanding of the reinforcing nature of a smile, a nod, a wink or an approving grunt. It is only to be hoped that psychologists do not gain the same reputation for phoney superficiality.
>
> The failure to recognise the difference between objectivism in measurement and objectivism in manipulation is central to the change which threatens to affect the clinical psychologist's role. It is ironic that just when research in psychotherapy is at last leading to some consistent picture of the kind of variables which seem therapeutically effective in human relationships—for example, warmth, empathy and genuineness (Traux & Carkhuff, 1967)—an increasing number of clinicians in this country are apparently uncritically espousing a consciously manipulative approach to patients and others which entails a radically different kind of relationship. Whether or not this kind of behavioural manipulation is successful is beside the point: what needs to be considered is whether one wishes to foster social organisation along these lines. Nobody but a psychological ostrich could deny that there is a difference between being smiled at genuinely

and being smiled at by someone who deliberately wishes to 'reinforce' one's behaviour. The most frightening thought of all is that, given the general population's gullibility in relation to modern technology, if this difference is denied often enough and categorically enough, conscious manipulation may become the norm. Societies can change, and social scientists can help to change them. They should perhaps be more aware than they are of their responsibilities in this respect, and of the contributions which they may unthinkingly be making to change.

The charge of Machiavellianism against the conscious and deliberate attempt to exercise these skills can be countered by the riposte that this is in fact how parents bring up children, how children and others interact in their groups and how people in a wide range of other contexts, in sales, service, the professions, and sport will influence others. What is described as genuineness is simply the highly expert and often unconscious exercise of these skills. The crucial ethical point is not whether or not skills should be used but to what end they should be used. If the aim is towards the humanisation of both patients and staff, if the aim is towards the enrichment of their day-to-day lives and towards the fulfilment of the potential of all of them working together to a common goal, then there is surely nothing less genuine in smiling to someone with a view to reinforcing appropriate behaviour on their part than there is in presenting genuine 'Largactil' tablets to someone who is genuinely emotionally disturbed. Nevertheless, Smail's main points are taken and it would be foolish to omit consideration of these issues in a general discussion on the role of the psychologist in an institution.

In any event, no clinical psychologist is going to undertake his functions, whether these be entirely professional, executive, or in social engineering, without due consideration of the kind of views expressed in the prologue to the 'Ethical Standards of Psychologists' of the American Psychological Association (1963). This should surely go some way to allaying Smail's anxiety. 'The psychologist believes in the dignity and worth of the individual human being. He is committed to increasing man's understanding of himself and others. While pursuing this endeavour, he protects the welfare of any person who may seek his services or of any subject, human or animal, that may be the object of his study. He does not use his profession or relationships, nor does he knowingly permit his own services to be used by others, for purposes inconsistent with these values. While demanding for himself freedom of enquiry and communication he accepts the responsibility this freedom confers, for competence where he claims it, for objectivity in the report of his findings, and for consideration of the best interests of his colleagues and of society'.

CHAPTER V

ASPECTS OF BODY IMAGE

It is pleasant and informative to start with a number of quotations, one of which is well enough known, the second of which may be a little surprising and the third of which, although unknown to most, may have a horrible relevance to a few. The first is from Robert Burns (1785):

> O wad some Pow'r the giftie gie us
> *To see oursels as others see us!*
> It wad frae monie a blunder free us
> An' foolish notion:
> What airs in dress an' gait wad lea'e us
> And ev'n Devotion!

Much of the writer's research on this general topic stems from that particular verse and attempts to operationalise it in practical form. The second is from Sir Cyril Burt (1937) and has already found a place in this book in spite of that recent fall from grace in some other respects. It is:

> It is a truism in psychology that the mechanism of the mind stands on a sensory-motor basis. The world outside can stimulate the mind only through one of the senses; and, in return, all that the greatest intellect can do is to contract a set of muscles and move a set of bony levers. The end product of every mental process is simply a muscular reaction.

It was that particular paragraph which developed the author's concern for the relationship between motor skill and human performance and our notions of what we are like as physical objects. Finally, there is a complete poem by Frederick Busch (1972) which illustrates in an interesting, allusive and evocative style the self-perceptions and cathexes of a typical comfort loving endomorph, psychologist or otherwise:

> WHAT THE BODY SAYS
>
> Bag of death I drag beneath my head
> he names his body, hauling It
> down the stairs to breakfast, propping the corpse up
> in his chair, naming, watching the bulge
> at the buttons he wears on his belly,

whinnying at how he curls and shimmies
to crawl from his car to walk upstairs to work,
where he names the life his mind athletically lopes in
while his body catches Its breath.

For lunch a public sandwich and a beer,
a smuggled Milky Way, Mars Bar up the sleeve
that curls round the 'Times'
(the people are spying on the President again)
and torpor at the torpid desk, like after sex
but pregnanter with hate for you know what,
the way It overflows the arms of the swivel chair
like sluggish oleomargarine, just melting nearly
on the move. He names It bag of death
and turns the page; snick like an ace,
the Mars Bar drops. The cards are on the table.

For dinner: everything. Then sneaky rice
from the pot's bottom, a tongue to the serving spoon,
a trembling at the television set as It
settles, like a giant landscape, for the long night:
he hears Its far-off rumblings, subterranean
gurgles of unknown dreadful moistnesses, the gradual
collapse of the surface onto the secrets beneath.

Breathing slyly, he names It again
Bag of death he's chained to,
names It, there is silence, the picture jumps,
the lights hiss, the room winks like an eye, he hates
himself from head to toe, he names It—Bag of death
—and there is silence in the flickering room
and then he hears It name him who is
head which hauls a sack of inconvenience through his life.
It whispers Bag of death.

Now although it might be thought that this sort of opening is a kind of *jeu d'esprit* which might more properly find its place in a middle class literary society, these quotations, nevertheless, at once embrace the peculiar quantitative and qualitative aspects of the 'self' as it is perceived by each of us—the vision and experience of our own body and identity as endorsed by our interaction with the environment and with other people. They also embrace the clear awareness that overt behaviour, often skilled, is determined at least in part by the accuracy of one's notion of what one is like as a physical object, with dimensions, properties and kinetic potential, and, finally, how we feel about our bodies emotionally, and consciously or unconsciously evaluate them.

The term 'body image' occurs with considerable regularity in texts and papers within the fields of psychiatry, neurology and psychology, often without much attempt to define it either theoretically or operationally. Frequently it is used in such a way as to suggest that not only has it explanatory value, but also that it may have some vague mediating influence on behaviour, as diverse as adapting to an amputated limb on the one hand or coping with a learning disability on the other.

Neurologists seem largely to understand body image as something which is disturbed, often by right parietal lobe malfunction but remark on it less frequently when it appears to be functioning well or normally. Psycho-analysts and dynamically oriented psychologists incorporate within the concept not only 'the body schema' of the neurologists, but also the whole range of learned experiences, attitudes and emotional cathexes which one's sense of identity, closely associated with one's body and its integrity, demands. Thirdly, there are the cognitively oriented psychologists whose concern is with the body as the object as well as the subject of perception and who would consider that, since the rules of perception of bodies and of non-body objects may not be the same, other theories must relate to their submissions about the habits of and determinants of body perception in man.

The first part of this chapter will give some of the theoretical background to past work on body image and related constructs. The second part will present some experimental evidence concerned particularly with the personal evaluative aspect of body image. For once the data are interesting not because they demonstrate differences between mentally subnormal and normal subjects, but because they *do not* when almost all other related data do.

Since people are so patently, and so literally, bound up in their own bodies, and since these are the instruments of so much higher nervous activity as well as the physical evidence of our very existence, it seems pertinent to ask whether body image might or might not have the unitary properties it is so often asserted to possess. Alternatively, the term should perhaps be used in a global way and taken more to subsume a number of subsidiary but overlapping concepts, each of which is concerned with particular aspects of body image. The writer (Clark, 1975) has already done this elsewhere in some detail and has demonstrated that the notion is certainly not a unitary construct, the factors comprising it being substantially different in content and structure between, for example, normal subjects and the handicapped. This will be touched on later.

The many connotations of the term 'body image' and the variety of contexts in which it has been used are at the root of most of the conceptual and some of the operational problems which it has presented. Smythies (1953) in a pertinent though philosophically oriented paper, considered that there was 'confusion in neurology and allied disciplines between the body image, the body schema, the body concept and the perceived body'. Thirty years later this confusion remains, but does not seem to have deterred, in the interim, a substantial number of writers from using the concept relatively freely in a global way and in a variety of contexts at differing levels of explanatory power. Curiously, it is when the concept is used to explain certain phenomena occurring in diseased, disturbed or traumatically damaged bodies that it has least ambiguity. It must be noted, however, that many body image phenomena observed by most normal people, may represent healthy psychophysiological responses and indicate no emotional or psychological disturbance whatsoever. Probably it is when differences among normals are discussed that the concept is used most loosely. Smythies (1953) has followed Reitman (1950) in indicating that arguments relevant to one set of data may be wrongfully transposed to provide most misleading conclusions when applied to another set of data, especially when other terms might better have been used. Our knowledge of body image when it is functioning normally in undamaged individuals may not necessarily be safely derived from our knowledge of body image or deficits in body image found in subjects who have been traumatically injured or who are pharmacologically disturbed.

In his work Smythies is most concerned with this difficulty as a philosophic one and he concerns himself primarily to distinguish what he terms the 'perceived body', the actual physical body and the body image. The perceived body he considers a term which should be applied 'to the somatic sensory field'. It is comprised of the totality of all somatic sensa available to inspection in any one moment. He points out that 'the perceived body is thus not the same thing as the physical body. The special inter-relations of parts of the perceived body reproduce those of the physical body because there is a system of signalling mechanisms between the two. When this signalling mechanism goes wrong, as in certain brain lesions, in mescaline intoxication, and schizophrenia, the behaviour of the perceived body may be quite different from that of the physical body, but follows exactly the state of the body image in the brain'. Smythies goes on to comment that the apparent size of the physical body is clearly very much larger than the perceived body which he sees as a function of cortical activity within the brain. He thus distinguishes the perceived body from the body image which he considers to be something greater than the perceived body in the sense that it is a spacial object which has both visual, mental and memory images bound up in it either of one's own or someone else's body. He is less concise in distinguishing between body image and body concept. Broadly speaking, the distinction is that the former is contributed to by a knowledge of bodies generally, including other persons' bodies, whereas Smythies sees the latter as depending on ego differentiation and self-knowledge only. As he says, 'the term body concept properly describes the constellation of memories and beliefs we each possess concerning our own physical bodies. Both body image and body concept are, of course, fluid creations neither of them being always accurate since they are affected by wishes, by pride, by natural change with experience and ageing.

'Disparities between the perceived body and the physical body are clearly exemplified by the phantom limb phenomena. Yet the individual will know that he has only one physical leg perhaps and his body concept as an intellectually structured phenomenon is unaffected although the phantom will continue to puzzle and sometimes distress him. In the same way, in autotopagnosia there is a pure disorder of perception whereby the perceived body has parts missing while in anosognosia there is a concomitant disorder of the body concept. In such conditions the physical body remains intact and the perceived body may have one entire side destroyed by the cerebral lesion. In the first case the patient may answer correctly such questions as "How many legs have you?", whereas in the second the patient may answer incorrectly, showing a disorder of the body concept'.

Parallel to this conceptual system available to consciousness and relating to our physical structure, it can be considered that there is a system of subconscious knowledge of experience stored up belonging to the system described by Sherrington (1940) as 'the motor individual'. This is much more like the 'body schema' as defined by Head & Holmes (1911) and again by Head (1926) and can be thought of as a purely physiological mechanism operating outside consciousness and related to the sensory cortex. Smythies describes it as 'the great system of cerebral mechanisms', responsible for posture, automatic movements and the co-ordination of voluntary movement 'the activity of which goes on below "the threshold of consciousness", or, better, outside perceptual space, without our knowing any more about it than that our actions are carried out efficiently. It possesses the totality of information about the state of the physical body and its environment'. Head & Holmes (1911) define the *body schema* as 'the fundamental standard against which all postural changes are measured', and when they develop this idea at a later time they add, ' ... in addition to its function as an organ for local attention, the sensory cortex is also the storehouse for past impressions. They may rise into consciousness as images, but more often, as in the case of spacial impressions, remain outside central consciousness. Here they form organised models of ourselves which may be termed "schemata". Such schemata modify the impressions produced by incoming sensory impulses in such a way that the final sensations of position, or of locality, rise into consciousness charged with a relation to something that has happened before'.

Ritchie-Russell (1958) was also concerned with the mediating effect of the body schema on motor action. Effective actions such as, for example, scratching one's back, feeding, dressing, jumping or driving a car or a golf ball can only be carried out against a developed, if sub-conscious, awareness of the body's physical and kinetic characteristics and position in space. His definition was entirely operational: 'that which makes it possible for appropriate bodily movements to be performed in relation to afferent stimuli'.

Thus body schema can be thought of as being constantly updated by the input resulting from further movements of the body whether these be active or passive. The schema in this sense then is an integrated resultant of past sensory experience and a unity deriving from these experiences together with current sensations organised in the sensory cortex. Such a schema functioning outside central consciousness can be considered to modify impressions of incoming sensory impulses for their localisation on the body surface and also makes possible intricate and delicate motor activities through the constant relationship of the body to other objects. As Kolb (1959) puts it, 'thus Head conceptualised in the area of sensory motor functioning, a postural model of the body, which brings about the possibility of projecting the recognition of posture, movement, and locality beyond the limits of the body to the ends of instruments held in the hand or operated by the body. Anything which participates in movement of the body was seen as added to the postural model and as becoming a part of the body schema'.

Smythies (1953) finds it hard to see how the acceptance of the visual component of body image can do other than confuse the use of the concept and certainly he would challenge the classical definition of the body image by Schilder (1950): 'The image of the human body means the picture of our own body that we form in our mind, that is to say, the way in which the body appears to ourselves'. Smythies feels that this sentence refers too much to a visual image only and that the second part of the sentence is full of ambiguities. However, Schilder goes on later: 'There are sensations which are given to us. We see part of the body surface. We have tactile, thermal, pain impressions. There are sensations coming from the muscles and their sheaths, indicating the deformation of the muscles; and sensations coming from the viscera. Beyond that there is the immediate experience that there is a unity of the body. This unity is perceived, yet it is more than a perception. We call it a schema of our body or body schema ... '. Smythies's view is that all the sensa outlined in the above passage, with the exception of the visual, make up at any instant what he would describe as the perceived body. Schilder later acknowledges the body schema of Head emphasizing the knowledge of position of the body and its postural model.

One summing up of the above views is best represented by a straightforward quotation from Smythies's (1953) paper. 'The perceived body is directly experienced inside central consciousness. The existence of even the individual observer's own physical body is inferred. The term body image should be reversed to describe a visual, mental, or memory image of a human body. Body images are experienced. The constant visual imagery relating to the body and parts of the body associated with movement and sensation is integrated, largely by the subconscious system of cerebral mechanisms, into the unitary function of the human organism. The term body schema should only be used in its original sense. It is part of the subconscious mind and thus its presence is inferred. The body concept is a conceptual constellation and it depends largely on the proper function of the relevant memory mechanisms'. A recent critical review of some of these usages and constructs has been that of Poeck & Orgass (1971).

Perhaps the best general definition of body image in the sense that it will be used in this chapter is that of Witkin et al. (1962) where they describe it as 'the systematic impression an individual has of his body, cognitive and affective, conscious and unconscious, formed in the process of growing up'. This has the merit of incorporating the 'perceived body' notions of Smythies, the more composite concept of Schilder, and of accepting too that the structuring of perception and the development of feelings and emotions in relation to the body itself and its parts will play their part in modifying the construct. Moverover, the fact that they accept both conscious and unconscious components allows the incorporation of 'schemata' in Head's sense and, finally, there is an acceptance of modification and adaptation of the body image with development and maturation. Witkin (1965), interestingly, sees the body concept as preceding the body image developmentally in that he recognises the child's growing capacity to learn not only his body boundaries but also that the body has various parts and processes, discrete yet interrelated and put together in a definite structure. As the child recognises this in itself and in others it is building up a concept of the body reflected in its use of language and in drawing, for example, which acts as an organising principle for perception, especially, in Witkin's view, when stimulus conditions for body perception are indefinite.

As important as any of the ideas incorporated in Witkin's definition is the developmental view which would be particularly supported by both Piaget (1952) and Merleau-Ponty (1962). It has always, for example, been Piaget's view that development of the body image runs parallel with sensory motor development, reflecting the importance of movement activity and with its related kinaesthetic feedback. The latter writer also considers that the development of personal differentiation is an important aspect of perceptual growth although he does not really discriminate between the tems of body boundary and body image except to suggest that the realisation of the former is necessary for the latter. The skin, of course, forms the ultimate body boundary and it is at this interface between body and external environment that the exchange of information takes place. There is a sense therefore in which body image can be seen as being built up as a result of information processing by the organism of data deriving from both the internal and external environments. This information may include data from the external environment which is not the result of the individual's own actions (exafferent) together with (re-afferent) data which is the result of his own actions.

The literature is parsimonious in its specific references to the problems of body image in the mentally subnormal. Ajuriaguerra (1965) comments that 'an arrest of the development of operational functions, such as is seen in oligophrenia ... will produce disturbances essentially in body representation as well as in constructive praxias and other operational activities'. Wapner & Werner (1965), however, stress the role of the environmental context in perception of our own bodies. They found from their experiments that subjects' estimates of their own dimensions were smaller when made in a confined space as against when made in a wide open space. Thus they take the view that 'perception of body space and perception of external space are not independent, but rather interact intimately'. The same writers go on to comment on how, on the evidence of other work (Werner, 1940; Wapner & Werner, 1957; Werner & Kaplan, 1963; Wapner, 1964a, 1964b) they assume on developmental principles that the boundary between body space and outside space is lessened with lower developmental status and consequently groups such as the mentally subnormal should overestimate apparent body dimensions, especially head width. They reason that schizophrenics and normal adults under primitivising drugs should demonstrate the same phenomenon. In more recent literature (Maloney, Ball & Edgar, 1970; Kephart, 1960) all to some extent reflect the quotation of Burt's that the writer remarked on at the outset of the chapter in that they propose that there will be beneficial effects of sensory motor training on the development of body image in the mentally subnormal. Unfortunately, these authors tended to measure body image using individual tests of unknown validity.

As a general rule, Benton (1955a), Fink, Greene & Bender (1953), together with a number of others, have demonstrated that body schema deficits tend to be associated with retarded intellectual functioning. However, these studies have been carried out only with children. The writer (Clark, 1975) has reviewed elsewhere in detail some of the work reported in this area but very little has been done with adult populations in particular and of that some is conflicting in its evidence about body image in mentally subnormals. This is again because so many different operational definitions of body image have been adopted, with consequent uncertainty about general validity. Broad conclusions from the available literature might be as follows. First, for an effectively differentiated body image to be developed, both central nervous system and peripheral neural structures and functioning must be intact. The role of bodily habitus is less clear. Second, the mentally subnormal may be thought of as having difficulty, for a variety of reasons, in progressing developmentally beyond the sensory motor or pre-operational stage of cognitive growth and consequently as having less mature cognitive styles than normals together with more misperceptions and faulty classifications of experience. It could be predicted accordingly that the body image concept in the mentally subnormal would be less well developed when assessed by a variety of standard tests. More particularly, retardates might be expected to over-estimate certain, but not all, body dimensions and to be unsure of body boundaries. Motor/perceptual tests are likely to be more reliable than verbal/questionnaire type tests, especially if instructions can be simple and not verbally complicated. Some measures such as the 'barrier' and 'Penetration' scores of Fisher & Cleveland (1958) appear to be too contaminated by intelligence and general social/cultural competence to be valid body image measures in the retarded population and there is evidence that retardates may establish socially preferred body images so that certain physical structural types carry different emotional loadings, just as they do for normal subjects. On the whole, however, the literature contributes little to the proposition that low intelligence has little effect on the affective/evaluative aspect of body image.

If this is the background of thinking about body image in the general literature, what in fact can be discovered experimentally? Attention on this occasion will be drawn only to some experimental findings from a larger study by the author (Clark, 1975). These will be concerned to demonstrate not only that there is no unitary construct of body image, but also that the factorial structure of body image shows intelligence-related differences. Within that general context, however, there are a number of individual test results which show no significant differences between the mentally subnormal and normal subjects, and it is these which are now reported.

Some outline of the general strategy of the research, however, is required to put these in their setting. As has been indicated above, body image has, in the past, usually been measured in the reported literature using only one or at best two tests such as Benton's Ear, Hand and Eye Test, a variety of Body Size Estimation tests such as used by Shontz (1969) or Fisher & Cleveland's Barrier and Penetration variables from the Holtzman or Rorschach Ink Blot techniques. The literature was searched for a variety of such tests and, to the resulting melange of procedures were added a number of measures, designed by the writer (Clark, 1975) either as refinements of previously used test techniques or as techniques which appeared to have face value as measures of body or self perception at either a visual, tactual or conceptual level. As a result of this, some 30 different measures were used for factor analytic purposes, deriving from some 15 different test operations. These tests included three of intelligence, the Progressive Matrices, the Peabody Picture Vocabulary Test and the Goodenough Harris Draw a Person Test. From the latter, for example, two derived measures were developed, one a Dimensional Index representing the size of drawing produced on a standard format paper, and two, a Body Image Disturbance scale which derived originally from work by Machover (1949) and Fisher (1959), and is a technique of rating particular anomalous features in a drawing, such as the presence of transparencies, the lack of limbs, the drawing of a nude figure, asymmetries, erasures, bizarre anatomical features and so forth. Others included the Secord & Jourard (1953) Body Cathexis Scale, Two-Point Threshold, the Witkin Rod and Frame Test, a Finger Apposition Test developed by the writer, and two major test procedures, each giving rise to a number of measures especially developed for the research, involving a Body Distorting Mirror on the one hand, and Body Size Estimation apparatus on the other. Other aspects of the research took account of relationships between motor skill and body image and utilised a series of tests of the former, over and above the drawing test, such as Pursuit Rotor performance, Reaction Time to auditory and visual stimuli, a Mirror Tracking test with a number of measures deriving from it, a Motor Steadiness test and so forth.

Although further data are still being accumulated, the initial populations were of 50 moderate subnormals, 25 of each sex, matched with 50 normals for age, sex, socio-economic level and physical integrity. It is perhaps worth noting in passing that it is remarkably difficult to find a population who are borderline subnormals or worse and who at the same time do not have significant skeletal or sensory defects (other than eyesight corrected by wearing glasses) or who are free from obvious central nervous system disorder. The introduction of uncontrolled variables of that sort might certainly have made the interpretation of the findings overwhelmingly difficult but it may well be that in the event greater clarification of some of the constructs emerging from the research may be achieved by selectively using particular skeletally or CNS disrupted samples. Among the experimental subjects the mean ages of the male and female groups were 25.84, standard deviation 8.39 and 26.08, standard deviation 9.18 respectively, and in the case of the control groups, males had a mean age of 25.84, SD 7.97, and females a mean age of 25.80, SD 9.06. With regard to intelligence, the experimental males had a mean IQ of 68.56, SD 8.78, the females 63.84, SD 8.92 whereas the control population mean IQ male was 110.88, SD 12.20, and females 113.20, SD 10.72. There were no significant differences in age, nor were there significant sex differences.

Many of the test results, which will not be quoted in this paper, showed, as expected, fairly massive differences in score distributions between subnormal and normal subjects, especially those which might be taken to represent aspects of *body schema* after Sherrington or Head & Holmes. Among these were the Two Point Threshold measurement, the Body Disturbance Index from the drawing test, Finger Apposition test, and to a lesser extent, the Rod and Frame test. Estimates of Body Size in both light and dark conditions also showed very significant differences, although whether these related more to aspects of body percept or were contaminated by intelligence factors, is more open to debate. The tests which, however, showed similar score distributions in normal and subnormal subjects were the figure drawing Dimensional Index, the Secord Jourard Body Cathexis Scale scores and some scores derived from the Body Distorting Mirror technique. Brief descriptions of these latter tests now follow.

The Goodenough Harris DAP Test was initially introduced in the research programme, not only because it contributed to an overall assessment of intelligence but also because many researchers in the body image field have used it, partly as a projective device, but also as a measure of expressive motor behaviour of a more specific kind. For example, two previous factor analytic studies of the drawing test indicated subsidiary factors of a size element (Nichols & Strumpfer, 1962) and a factor discriminated by these authors as one concerned with defence and constriction. In a second study by Adler (1970) a second factor of size and placement seemed to confirm Nichols & Strumpfer's work. Quite apart from the reliability coefficients so far as intelligence measurement is concerned, inter-judge reliabilities tended to be around 0.52 and test/retest reliabilities up to 0.85 for the size element in figure drawings. The test/retest reliability for subjects in the writer's own research was found to be 0.79. The *Dimensional Index* itself was arrived at by measuring in millimetres the longest axis of the drawing from the top of the head, including hair, to the tips of the toes or soles of the feet as the case may be, and then taking a similar measure at right angles to that axis across the resultant widest part of the drawing. The Dimensional Index was the square root of the product of these two dimensions. This, therefore, is a measure of the size of the drawing in the sense that area rather than height is being assessed and the technique accords more with the procedures adopted in the better studies just quoted. It seems not unlikely from these studies that size of drawing thus represented might relate to a factor such as disinhibition, or behavioural extravagance, while micrographic drawings could be taken complementarily to reflect inhibitedness, constriction of personal response pattern, or a lowering of self-esteem, or withdrawal and hesitancy, perhaps even of higher anxiety levels (Machover, 1949; Hammer, 1958; Gray & Pepitone, 1964 and Lakin, 1960).

In their original paper on the topic of *Body Cathexis*, Secord & Jourard (1953) commented that the one object which is ever present in an individual's personal world is his body and that remarkably little attention had been paid in personality theory, especially to the individual's attitudes to it. At the time they thought that body cathexis, as they understood it, was specifically related to the self concept, although probably a separate aspect of the latter. In particular, they sought to test the hypothesis that feelings about the body were tantamount to feelings about the self, and both were appraised by similar scales; second, that negative feelings about the body tended to be associated with anxiety in the form of undue concern with pain, disease or injury; and third, that negative feelings about the body could be associated with feelings of insecurity involving the self. In brief, their work confirmed these hypotheses and Johnson (1956) and Gunderson & Johnson (1965) later confirmed the correlations between body and self cathexis which Secord & Jourard (1953) had reported.

The Body Cathexis Scale is composed of 46 items which the subject rates on a five-point basis, ranging from strong positive to strong negative feelings. Each item of the scale which could be a body part or function was followed by numbers 1 to 5 and the subject was asked to rate whether in respect of the body part or function listed, they had: (1) strong feelings and they wished change could somehow be made, (2) don't like but can put up with, (3) have no particular feelings one way or the other, (4) am satisfied or (5) consider myself fortunate. It is interesting to note at this point that Jourard & Secord in a later study in 1955 concerned themselves with the relationship of the Body Cathexis Scale scores to discrepancies between the subjects' estimates of the ideal sizes for given body parts and the actual sizes they ascribe to these parts. There were significant indications that the greater the discrepancy between estimated ideal and estimated size for certain body dimensions, the more negative was the cathexis rating assigned. In the case of the research reported, a total score was used by simply summating the ratings accorded to each item, since this gave a wider dispersion of integer scores. The original authors divided their total score by 46 (i.e. the number of items). They quoted reliability coefficients on test/retest of from 0.78 to 0.83. The normative data supplied by the authors suggests that the mean total score of males is 157.78, SD 15.5 and of females 159.16, SD 18.95.

Body distorting mirror technique takes its origins from early work by Wittreich & Radcliffe (1955) who had asked subjects to stand in front of a large mirror and to describe themselves when either wearing or not wearing aniseikonic lenses. A year later Schneiderman (1956) had attempted to measure self estimation of the facial reflection in a small calibrated flexible mirror, 20 inches square, contained in a frame with ½ inch deep channels within which the mirror was bent by a set of screws. Later still Traub & Orbach (1964) developed Schneiderman's technique and used a somewhat larger mirror.

The apparatus developed by the writer consists of a sheet of perspex some 48 inches by 18 inches of a resilience such that it bends in cylindrical section rather than in parabolic or hyperbolic section when forces are applied to the ends. The mirror was vacuum plated with aluminium since any other technique had been found either to crease, crinkle or crack the mirroring of the silver nitrate which is the more normal technique. The bending of the mirror was adjusted by electric motors through gear-boxes which drove screwed rods, passing through clamped bodies holding the edges of the mirror. The amount of distortion from a plane surface which was applied to the mirror was measured in arbitrary units by small rotary indicators such as are found in tape recorder counters. Only one dimension was varied at a time and symmetrical distortions were used. The experimenter controlled the electric motors by a series of switches and the subject was presented with a particularly distorted image as he stood some 5ft 6ins from the apparatus in a neutrally draped room with minimal visual cues. The subject was then asked to watch the mirror as the experimenter reduced its distortion and to say "Stop" as soon as he felt that a true image of himself appeared. Both ascending and descending measures were taken, with a counterbalanced design, so that alternate subjects started from a different end point. Initially, five runs were carried out and a mean performance taken as the measure. In later studies, however, only two runs were taken since reliabilities are shown to be very high on this apparatus (from 0.716 to 0.978 test/retest and split half).

The subject could be presented, therefore, with four separate problems; one in which he was seen to be taller than he is, one in which he appeared to be shorter, one in which he appeared to be fatter and one in which he appeared to be thinner. The point at which the mirror was stopped by the subject on ascending and descending measures was noted and the mean of those two readings was taken as his midpoint representation in that dimension. The arrangement of the counters was such that a score of 20 on the unit counter represented an absolutely plane surface in the mirror and consequently a veridical image. It can be seen that the difference between the two scores on ascending and descending runs represents the extent of the range of images of oneself which a given subject might find acceptable. If the midpoint of these is at the point scoring 20 (when the subject is reflected by a plane surface) this could be thought of as a veridical representation but if the midpoint is elsewhere then that measures the deviation from veridicality of the subject's representation of himself. In the same way, the range of acceptable scores could be very narrow or very large.

In order to clarify whether the process of representing one's own body visually in this matter was equivalent to representing a non-body object, a randomly shaped piece of hardboard having approximately similar overall area to a subject's torso was mounted on a stand and placed in such a position that the subject could see it reflected in the mirror without seeing his or her own reflection, and also so that the optical distance from the subject's eye to the object was as near as possible to the overall distance from the subject's eye to the surface of the mirror to the object. Similar measures were taken with the subject representing this neutral object.

On the day of testing, and before the distorting mirror or body size estimate tasks were presented, all subjects were engaged in casual conversation in which care was taken to ask, among other questions, in the same order, the following questions: 'Do you know what you look like?', 'Would you like to be different in any way?'. If the latter question was answered in the affirmative the following questions 'Would you like to be either taller or shorter than you are?' or 'Would you like to be either fatter or thinner than you are?' were asked.

Results

The following tables present the results on these three tests.

There are the usual signs of fairly wide scatter in subnormal populations in the Dimensional Index distributions. But it is remarkable that there are no significant differences in mean size across all the subgroups. This is of particular interest in the light of the fact that the intelligence measures derived from the same drawings showed massive differences. Such a phenomenon is, of course, entirely in keeping with the views put forward by both Nichols and Strumpfer (1962) and Adler (1970) indicating that the second factor determining performance in a drawing test was one representing size as distinct from the first factor of intellectual competence.

TABLE 1: *Body Distortion Mirror Task: Range—Body Length*

Interval*	Group 1 Male Exp	Group 2 Male Con	Group 3 Fem Exp	Group 4 Fem Con
24.000)				
22.000)			*	
20.000)				
18.000)			*	
16.000)	*			
14.000)	***	**	**	*
12.000)	*	**	**	*
10.000)	*	***	****	****
8.000)	****	*	****	*****
6.000)	****	*****	**	**
4.000)	***	***	*	**
2.000)	****	**	*	********
0.000)	****	*******	*******	**
Mean	6.800	5.880	7.880	6.160
SD	4.805	4.576	6.146	3.955
N	25.	25.	25.	25.

All Groups)	Mean	6.6800	Maximum	22.0000
Combined)	SD	4.9213	Minimum	0.0000

	Sum of Squares	DF	Mean Square	F Ratio
Between	59.1145	3	19.7048	0.8089
Within	2338.6333	96	24.3608	
Total	2397.7478	99		

*Printed interval designations are lower limits of class intervals

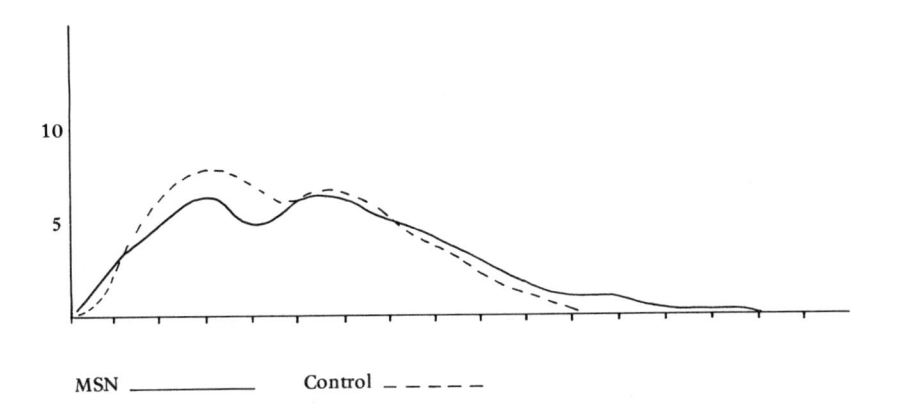

MSN ─────── Control ─ ─ ─ ─

TABLE 2: *Body Distorting Mirror Task: Midpoint—Body Length*

	Group 1 Male Exp	Group 2 Male Con	Group 3 Fem Exp	Group 4 Fem Con
Interval*				
30.000)				
27.000)	**			
24.000)			*	
21.000)	*		*	***
18.000)	*******	******	********	*****
15.000)	******	********	*******	********
12.000)	****	*****	*****	******
9.000)	*****	*****	***	**
6.000)				*
3.000)				
0.000)		*		
−3.000)				
−6.000)				
Mean	15.960	14.080	16.200	15.640
SD	5.192	4.182	3.651	3.718
N	25.	25.	25.	25.

| All Groups) | Mean | 15.4700 | Maximum | 28.0000 |
| Combined) | SD | 4.2485 | Minimum | 1.0000 |

	Sum of Squares	DF	Mean Square	F Ratio
Between	68.3457	3	22.7819	1.2726
Within	1718.5537	96	17.9016	
Total	1786.8994	99		

*Printed interval designations are lower limits of class intervals

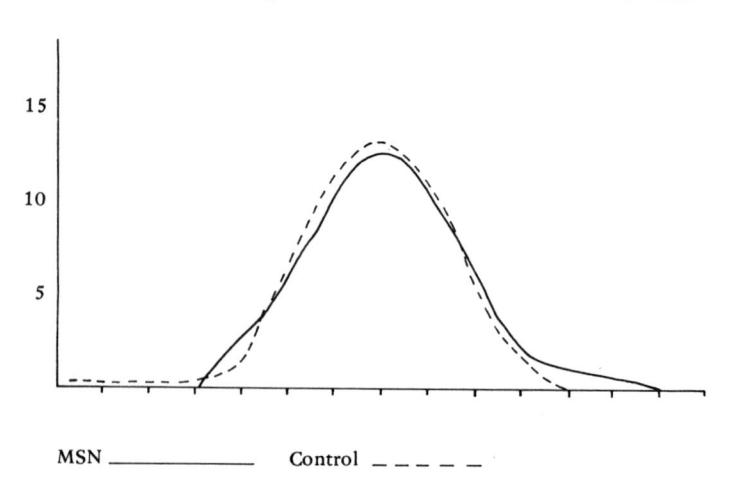

MSN ———— Control − − − − −

TABLE 3: Dimensional Index

	Group 1 Male Exp	Group 2 Male Con	Group 3 Fem Exp	Group 4 Fem Con
Interval*				
195.000)				
180.000)	**			
165.000)				
150.000)	*		**	
135.000)	*	*	*	**
120.000)	***	****	**	*
105.000)	****	******	**	********
90.000)	***	***	*******	********
75.000)	*****	*	******	****
60.000)	*	********	**	**
45.000)	***	*	**	
30.000)	**	*	*	
15.000)				
Mean	100.720	93.240	94.600	101.920
SD	40.503	28.950	30.654	19.910
N	25.	25.	25.	25.

All Groups)	Mean	97.6200	Maximum	187.0000
Combined)	SD	30.6430	Minimum	33.0000

	Sum of Squares	DF	Mean Square	F Ratio
Between	1408.8750	3	469.6250	0.4924
Within	91551.2500	96	953.6587	
Total	92960.1250	99		

*Printed interval designations are lower limits of class intervals

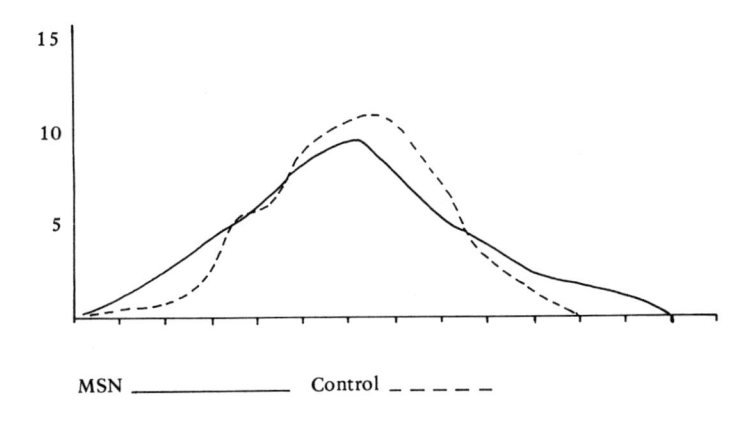

MSN —————— Control _ _ _ _ _

TABLE 4: Body Cathexis

	Group 1 Male Exp	Group 2 Male Con	Group 3 Fem Exp	Group 4 Fem Con
Interval*				
202.500)				
195.000)	*			
187.500)	*		*	
180.000)	**	*	*	
172.500)	*	**	***	**
165.000)	******	*******	**********	******
157.500)	***	*****	****	*******
150.000)	****	**	***	*****
142.500)	****	**	**	***
135.000)	**	****	*	
127.500)	*	*		*
120.000)				*
112.500)				
Mean	160.880	159.400	164.680	158.480
SD	17.025	13.865	11.499	12.965
N	25.	25.	25.	25.

All Groups)	Mean	160.8600	Maximum	198.0000
Combined)	SD	13.9761	Minimum	120.0000

	Sum of Squares	DF	Mean Square	F Ratio
Between	559.6055	3	186.5352	0.9536
Within	18778.2580	96	195.6068	
Total	19337.8630	99		

*Printed interval designations are lower limits of class intervals

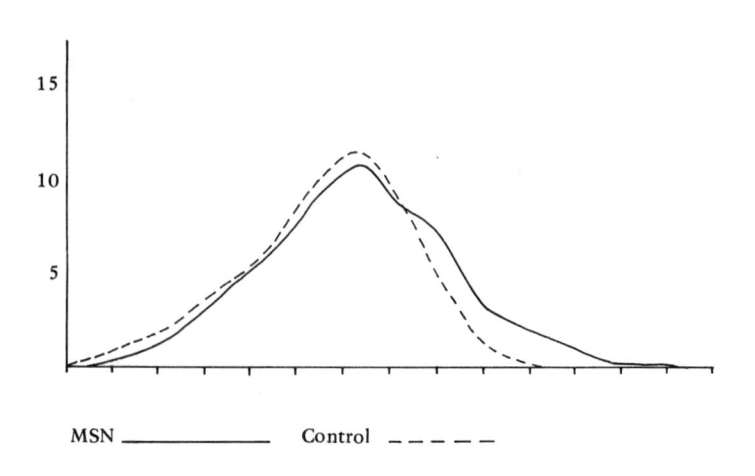

MSN ———— Control — — — —

Witkin, Dyke, Faterson, Goodenough & Karp (1962) have, of course, suggested that drawings of the human figure have provided indices of the degree of differentiation and a level of sophistication of the body image as a whole. It is clear, however, from their work that this differentiation concept is more closely related to cognitive development and if anything, to what we have described as body concept than it is to body image more generically defined. Because of the fragmentary nature of the studies, little of their work is definitive in this respect and perhaps the best and most succinct statement has been made by Silverstein & Robinson (1956) when they remark that 'the assumption that the physical body, the body image, and the drawn figure are in isomorphic relation remains as yet unjustified'.

Both Machover (1949) and Hammer (1958) considered that size of drawing was related to self esteem and energy level, with findings that high esteem subjects tended to draw larger figures. The study by Gray & Pepitone (1964) mentioned above experimentally manipulated self esteem by giving their subjects a series of personality tests, then reviewing the test results with the subjects in a way that would either enhance or deflate the subject's self esteem. Their findings were that high self esteem subjects' drawings tended to cover a greater area than low self esteem subjects' drawings. However, there is other evidence which suggests that the size of the figure reflects not only self esteem: it may reflect a more generalised anxiety. Koppitz (1966) for example, found that shy children drew small figures and Lewinsohn (1964) found that depressed subjects also tended to draw small figures. McHugh (1966) also found that children suffering from behaviour disturbances or tendencies to act out tended to draw larger figures than did neurotic or anxious children. If the IQ score from the figure drawing test shows significant differences between normals and subnormals in body concept, then the evaluative aspect of body image would appear to be different in kind and to be measured in at least one of its aspects by the Dimensional Index. What is perhaps more surprising is that in spite of the lack of sheer body size, in spite of other inadequacies and of poverty of intelligence, the distribution of self esteem as measured by this test is the same as it was for the controls in the subnormal group.

The Body Cathexis Scale scores show something similar. The *actual* body dimensions of the subnormal population in terms of height, for example, showed highly significant differences, particularly between female control and female experimental subjects. These differences were not so significant among the male controls and experimentals, but in spite of that and a general lack of prepossessingness in the subnormals, it was apparent that they did not themselves feel this but showed a normal range of acceptance or non-acceptance of body parts and function. Again the evaluative aspect of body image does not seem to be intelligence linked in the way that practically all other aspects of body schema and body concept are.

An evaluation of the significance of the Body Distorting Mirror results is more complex. This derives from the fact that intelligence linked differences do not appear when body height is being measured but do when body width is being measured. These differences disappear again when a neutral non-body object is being assessed. An incidental and fascinating result is that both normal and subnormal subjects tend to under-estimate their height on this task with no particular differences between subnormals and normals being shown in the *range* of images which are acceptable. There is, incidentally no apparent relationship between veridicality and whether subjects use a wide or narrow range of acceptable images. So far as body width is concerned, normal subjects are much more likely to be veridical and to use smaller ranges. In part this may be an artifact of the test apparatus but it is certainly not reflecting a generalised perceptual tendency since in the settings of the mirror to a neutral object all groups of subjects were veridical and all had similar range habits. Ranges on the neutral object were similarly rather smaller on all groups.

What seems to have been happening when subjects carried out the distorting mirror test was that they are presented with a configurational impression of themselves rather than having, as in some other tests, separate dimensions to estimate. It was, in fact, the visual equivalent of the evaluative tasks they were faced with in the Body Cathexis Scale completion but with a more directly visual component built into it rather than tapping what might have been described as body concept earlier in the paper. There is no ready explanation for why both normal and subnormal subjects should tend to depict themselves as rather shorter than they in fact were, except that some kind of experimental effect may have been operating to make them feel less secure and slightly to undervalue this particular dimension. It is certainly true that from data also collected in the research it appears to be more socially desirable to be taller rather than shorter in our culture. This seemed to be less true of being fatter or thinner and consequently no fixed effect showed up when that dimension was assessed using the mirror. More actually wished to be taller so they may have been a little self-conscious of seeming shortness and (as the data for width show) may have tended to depict themselves to exaggerate the deficit.

In conclusion, the writer's earlier research had certainly shown that there seemed to be merit in separating a number of components when talking about body image. In particular there are advantages in isolating the body schema with all the implications for what is going on in the neural substrate from the separate dimensional aspects of body parts which seem to be overdetermined by configurational and environmental contextual effects, and finally, from the evaluative or cathectic aspect of body perception. Consequently, different media for testing these distinct aspects of what has been mistakenly called body image are required. Mentally subnormal subjects do indeed show significant deficits in the first two aspects of body function or body perception which might underlie poorer motor or perceptual skill performance, but it seems that when presented with the tasks of attributing value to or deriving personal satisfaction and self esteem in regard to the whole or parts of one's body, the subnormal person is as much engaged and as accurately engaged in this as is anyone else. Clearly, social learning associated with the constant experience of actually being one's own body, using it in various tasks, having it described by others, having it valued, undervalued and overvalued by others, is something which is common to all of us and which must lead to a range of evaluative judgements about their bodies being made by individuals, independently of their intellectual capacity.

One implication of this is that we should pay as much attention in subnormal subjects as we accept in ourselves to body image enhancing characteristics like clothes, grooming, make-up, shoes and so on. We may be more helpful in this respect by eliciting what we can of the patient's views about his/her weak and strong points (as they see them) and by directing our counselling activities towards the moderation of self esteem—the reduction of too much as much as the boosting of too little—as well as by being thoughtful in our prescription of prosthetic appliances. At least two of the tests mentioned may give reliable indicators of the client's own current view of him/herself.

It may well be important to recognise this in dealing with our subnormal populations particularly, partly because it can then focus our efforts on those remedial activities which are particularly geared to dealing with those other aspects of body image which are, so to speak, in deficit, and which may have to be remedied using motor and perceptual re-educational techniques aimed at coping with an already subtly damaged neural substrate or skeletal structure, or at faulty habits of perception in general. Measures relating to the body schema or dimensional details of the body may help to detail this.

However, so far as the values attributed to one's own general visual appearance, to one's own attitudes to and feelings about oneself in human situations, or to one's self-satisfaction with one's physical structure are concerned, the recognition that there is the same dispersion of scores in normals and subnormals representing satisfaction, dissatisfaction and even complacency is something which may make us fear less for some aspects of the general emotional wellbeing of our patients. Indeed it may reassure us that the whole range of feelings and attitudes we ourselves can assimilate to our bodies and their functions is shared by subnormals even when many of us and them may be less than perfect in a variety of respects. Even the 'fatties' among us need not feel they are simply carrying around Frederick Busch's 'Bag of Death' but may have the liberated assurance of feeling that we in Secord & Jourard's terms warrant rating level 5 and in their words 'Consider ourselves fortunate'.

CHAPTER VI

PSYCHOTHERAPY: AN EXERCISE IN ECLECTICISM

The historical development of the study of mental subnormality shows clearly why psychotherapy and counselling have figured largely neither in the research nor in the clinical literature. This is in part because mental deficiency has generally been construed in terms of intellectual dysfunction measured by cognitive criteria and determined typically by an ability to perform various standardised tasks; or even, in simple terms, to achieve a given IQ. Partly too, it is because the first therapeutic approaches to the mentally retarded were fundamentally educational. They were directed towards improving achievement and attainment. The earliest popularly known work to remind us of this particularly is that of Itard (1932) on Victor, the Wild Boy of Aveyron, work which has recently brought into a new perspective the efforts of Ball (1971) and Kephart (1960, 1964) on developing sensory motor training programmes. Even their work, reviewed more fully in Chapter III, has however been linked very much more to the intellectual progress of the client than to his more general wellbeing involving personality functioning.

One is thus blinkered by the very term 'mental handicap' when it comes to taking a more differentiated look at the difficulties of those to whom the term is applied. Specious generalisation has occurred, with the result that all the difficulties and personal problems of the handicapped tend to be seen as a function of cognitive deficit. In spite of the rightly often repeated view that this special population is characterised by extreme heterogeneity, there is, because of the defining value of a cognitive measure like IQ, a deepseated bias among behavioural scientists towards the dangerous use of low IQ not only as a reification of a useful, but abstract, construct but also an an explanatory variable and, often, even as a criterion of therapeutic improvement. It is probably true that the majority of researches in this area of work during the past three decades have attempted to measure the effects of psychotherapy with the mentally handicapped in terms of IQ changes. It does not seem strange to these researchers that one seldom adopts such criteria of success in judging the effects of psychotherapy among normal or bright subjects. There is a suspicion therefore that because IQ so easily becomes a key variable in defining the population, a population different in so many other ways, a favourable change in intelligence is, in consequence, likely to be the most convincing evidence of more satisfactory personal functioning. The alternative, and equally humane possibility, that effective psychotherapy may make a dull person a more balanced, predictable or happier dull person seems somehow to have eluded these researchers. Sternlicht (1966) has expressed this point of view more fully by approving psychotherapy for 'the patient who feels his intellectual handicap'. These patients, especially when institutionalised, must need help and support in the face of social and familial rejection or restriction of common freedoms. They need it too to help them cope with their own impulsive disinhibition deriving from cortical inefficiency, with sexual restraints on their behaviour, with lack of ego-ideals together with the need to live easily within the inherent sociopsychological characteristics of a subnormal culture.

Nevertheless, in Beier's terms (1964) 'Behavioural disturbances in the mentally retarded are important as they reduce the retardate's effectiveness and efficiency and make him generally uncomfortable with himself and with others. The training and rehabilitation of the retarded can be interfered with or prevented as much by behavioural disorder as by intellectual deficit. In addition to these effects, behavioural disorders in the mentally retarded may (1) have profound and deleterious effects on the retardate's family and others who surround him, (2) result in the fixation of unnecessary infantile patterns of behaviour, and (3) eventuate in the development of more severe problems of adjustment, behavioural disturbances, or antisocial behaviour patterns requiring more extensive care and control in the future'. Such animadversions, coupled with the experience of most who have carried out any sustained work with the handicapped over a number of years confirm one in the view that psychotherapy with such subjects is indubitably relevant. Scrutiny of the literature, however, makes it apparent that but for a small rash of papers in the 1950s, many of which were gathered together by Stacey and De Martino (1957), and a few more isolated relatively modern contributions (Oliver, Simon & Clark, 1965; Craft, 1965; Sternlicht, 1966; Stone & Coughlan, 1973; and Gunzburg, 1974) there is relatively little sound research either into the technique or into the result of psychotherapy with such a sub-population.

In a recent volume of International Review of Research in Mental Retardation, the editor, Ellis (1981), very briefly reviews the content of the 10 volumes which have appeared over the past 15 years. These volumes purport to report most of the significant work of behavioural scientists in the field of mental deficiency during that time. Seventy-six chapters divide into 26 in the directly applied field and 50 concerned with research in the basic sciences related to the subject. Ellis remarks that he has exercised no editorial bias in the selection of subject matter and that consequently his policy reflects productivity in the various problem areas and in the basic/applied categories. It is significant that only one chapter (Sternlicht, 1966) in these 76 is concerned with the psychotherapy of the mentally defective. Disappointingly little, with the exception of Gunzburg's chapter in Clarke & Clarke (1974) has emerged from the literature since then.

Broadly speaking, this evidence of the unfashionable nature of psychotherapy with the mentally handicapped has derived from the tacit assumption that such subjcts could never benefit from any psychotherapeutic relationship because of its assumed dependence on the use of abstract concepts and verbal skills. Sarason (1953) was more explicit. 'The inability of such an individual to control or delay emotional expression, to seek and to accept socially appropriate substitute activities in the face of frustrations and restrictions, to view objectively the behaviour of others, to adjust or to want to adjust to the needs of others, to realise the sources and consequences of his behaviour, these have been considered the liabilities in the defective individual which make it difficult for him to comprehend and to adjust to the purposes of the psychotherapeutic interview. When one considers that language is almost the sole means of communication between the therapist and patient and that the defective individual has inordinate difficulty in using and comprehending verbal generalisations, it is not surprising that the usual psychotherapeutic interview has been viewed as unfeasible with such individuals'. It has also been thought that the inability of a subnormal individual to recognise that he has particular problems, accessible to psychotherapy, implies that he lacks a set of constructs within which his experience and relationships are contained. A third notion commonly adduced in the case of the mentally handicapped has been that of limited potential for growth. This is 'a bad fit' with the preconception of most trained psychotherapists that psychotherapy is concerned not only with the alleviation of symptoms but also with the process of personality growth and personal development. These views, while not totally refuted, can now be seen to be overly restricting and pessimistic by psychotherapists whose experience has taken them into the lush fields of non-verbal communication, paralinguistics, and operant conditioning as well as into the heavily over-grazed meadows of traditional dynamic psychotherapy.

Perhaps the fact that so much psychotherapy was psycho-analytic in type in the 1920s and 1930s accounts for the fact that between the early work of Itard and occasional papers such as that of Chidester & Menninger (1936) almost nothing concerning the psychotherapy of the subnormal was published. Nevertheless, a good deal was going on in the form of rehabilitation and training within institutions and there was, if not a dramatic, at least a steady improvement in general cultural attitudes to the subnormal, perhaps more particularly with the borderline and so-called 'high grade' subnormal. The first signs of a greater flexibility of approach and a willingness to accept techniques other than the purely verbal were hinted at by the work of Heiser (1951, 1954) on the results of psychotherapy in a residential school for the retarded. No less a figure than Carl Rogers (1951), too, commenting on his own explorations with particular techniques of client centred therapy, remarked that 'several years ago the theory of therapy seemed best phrased in terms of the development of verbalised insight. This type of formulation seems to us today to fall far short of explaining all the phenomena of therapy, and hence occupies a relatively small place in our current thinking'.

The move away from the requirement to cope with abstract constructs and fluent verbalisation was further hastened by Maslow (1954) who firmly expressed the view that there were at least six main ways in which psychotherapy could be seen to take place. First, by expression (through act completion, release, or catharsis), second, by basic need gratification (giving support, reassurance, protection, love or respect); third, by removing threat (protection, good social, political and economic conditions); fourth, by improving insight, knowledge and understanding; fifth, by suggestion or authority, and sixth, by positive self-actualisation, individuation or growth. 'It is probable', he said, 'that all systems of psychotherapy use all these basic medicines in varying proportions'. Stacey & De Martino (1957) expressed the view that while all of these were applicable to some extent in the therapy of the mentally retarded, in most instances, particularly with the institutionalised retardate, therapy probably occurs most often through expression (catharsis) and basic need gratification. It was their view that psychotherapy gave the handicapped person an unparalleled opportunity for giving uninhibited expression to various pent up grievances, feelings of frustration, hostility, aggression, fantasies, hopes and aspirations. In addition, it gave them opportunities to experience not only the need for attention and affection but also some gratification of this and could mitigate their strong feelings of insecurity, anxiety, rejection and isolation.

In discussing these issues, it is important to define what is meant here by 'mentally handicapped'. Later, some attempt to define what is meant by 'psychotherapy' in the same context will also be made.

A useful starting point is given by the American Association of Mental Deficiency which has defined mental retardation as 'sub-average general intellectual functioning which originates during the developmental period and is associated with impairment in adaptive behaviour' (Heber, 1961). How far sub-average is a tolerable term in this context is, however, in more dispute on this side of the Atlantic. The 1959 Mental Health Act in England does incorporate subnormal intelligence as a defining characteristic of mental deficiency but the corresponding 1960 Scottish Act does not. One important point about the American definition is that it refers particularly to the *current* status of the individual. It also goes further in defining what 'sub-average' means, taking this to refer to a performance of more than one standard deviation below the population mean in terms of general intellectual functioning as measured by objective tests. Just as British authorities have been concerned that the handicapped should not be exploited or be a danger to themselves or others, so also the Americans have tended to see poor social adjustment as a particularly important qualifying condition at the adult level. Social adjustment is assessed in terms of the degree to which the individual is able to maintain himself independently in the community, and possibly in gainful employment, as well as his ability to meet and conform to other personal and social responsibilities and standards set by the community. A movement towards precision in criteria of such behaviours is currently under way but has yet to be properly fulfilled in psychometric terms.

For practical purposes here, however, I adopt a criterion of minus two standard deviations of the IQ distribution rather than one. The population under discussion will therefore be one where the upper limits of IQ are likely to be 70 and the lower around 50 to 45. Inevitably because of social and health policies, those subjects who are relatively brighter on this limited spectrum will almost inevitably have a number of personal and social adjustment problems in addition to their dull intelligence. At the lower end of the spectrum persons will have failed to develop certain adaptive behaviours rather than having maladaptations. The preoccupation of the therapist with the lower intelligence group will be towards the reduction of behavioural deficit and will be, with the more intelligent group, the reduction of maladaptive behaviours and the substitution of more socially acceptable behaviours. Feelings of personal wellbeing on the part of the subject would, however, be considered as equally appropriate and cognate outcomes of successful psychotherapy.

There is little evidence in the literature or from clinical experience that skeletal or sensory defects in the subnormal need automatically rule them out of psychotherapy. These defects may, however, determine the nature of the psychotherapy to be used and whether the subject is treated individually or in a group. Attentional deficits of great severity and the very limited information processing capacity or general capacity of subjects of IQ under 40 do, however, normally preclude a psychotherapeutic approach. More will be said later, however, about criteria for selection for psychotherapy.

In general, there is little to be learned from the early literature about the nature of psychotherapy with the handicapped. Not only does it on the whole tend to be poorly defined, but, generally speaking, criteria in the literature up to the 1960s are extremely naive, procedures are poorly described, goals are seldom illustrated or the specification of these explained, and curiously, there is relatively little discussion of the nature of the task itself. English & English (1958) have defined 'psychotherapy' as 'the use of any psychological technique in the treatment of mental disorders or maladjustments'. But even the use of terms like 'psychological technique' tend to be vague and imprecise. This is not helped by the view expressed by Gunzburg (1974) that there is a good argument for the view that almost all activities indulged in with the mentally retarded which are aimed at improving their functioning in any respect whatsoever, are psychotherapeutic in nature in the sense that they do not directly depend on chemotherapy nor on physical treatments such as physiotherapy. It is true also that the use of many adjuvant techniques can predetermine the setting in which psychotherapy takes place. There is no reason at all why psychotherapy cannot be administered in an occupational training unit while the subject is working on rug making or woodwork just as much as it might be carried on in a ward or counselling room. However, the meaning of psychotherapy I have adopted here will follow that outlined by Gunzburg and will be characterised by three features: the systematic, regular and planned application of psychological techniques by a trained person; a consistent effort to establish interpersonal relationships for the purpose of ameliorating personal and social problems; and an attempt to assess and measure objectively the effectiveness of the psychotherapeutic procedures.

Two further features are perhaps worth commenting on in this context. The first is that unlike most other clients for psychotherapy presenting at, for example, general psychiatric out-patient clinics or to psychologists and psychiatrists via general practitioners or private practice, clients who are mentally handicapped tend not so much to *present themselves* for treatment as to be *chosen* for treatment by the specialists themselves. While a few will present themselves actively and will produce a variety of *cris de coeur* which instigate treatment, the vast majority are selected sometimes for incidental reasons from among their peers often on rather arbitrary grounds. To that extent they are the recipients of psychotherapy, willy nilly, rather than active collaborators in the venture.

The second feature of psychotherapy with the mentally handicapped is that although a few will be dealt with as individuals at out-patient clinics or in a domiciliary context, the vast bulk of experience of personnel in this field has been of psychotherapy with *groups* and *within institutions*. Anyone even remotely familiar with the works of Russell Barton (1961) and Goffman (1961) will be aware that, not infrequently, the institution is as much the cause and creator of a disturbance in personality malfunctioning as are pressures within the individual subject. In consequence, many aspects of psychotherapy could be concerned with minimising 'institutionalisation' in the sense that Goffman (1961) or Stanton & Schwartz (1954) use it, as well as furthering the personal development, reduction of distress and symptomatology of the subject. In elaboration of the definition of psychotherapy above, the planned application of psychological techniques is likely to include some techniques which are perhaps not commonly thought of as psychotherapeutic. Incentive schemes, occupational therapy programmes and some aspects of behaviour modification might fall within this rubric. Nevertheless these terms do suggest that the task is ongoing, that it sets itself systematic targets and procedures and that it is wholly planned and developed with an insightful awareness of the kinds of interactions that are appropriate at a given stage in the treatment. Secondly, the important view that the task is one in which interpersonal relationships are used constructively has never been in doubt. Even the mentally handicapped down to the levels under discussion are capable of a wide range of normal human emotions and capable of forming some quite persisting personal relationships. The third point made in our definition is perhaps less important for the practising therapist and more for his colleagues who observe him. This is the attempt to assess and measure objectively not only the outcome of the therapist's endeavours but to scrutinise in detail the nature of the process as it occurs.

Finally, if we accept that for the moment the psychotherapist's task would be to improve the ill-defined variable of personal adjustment in his client, to improve chronic under-achieving or to modify behaviours which are essentially unproductive, disruptive, asocial or even antisocial, then what is the extent of the need for psychotherapy in this special population. That question may be difficult to answer since, in the case of many of the behaviours listed above, the client may not even be aware that they are problems until the implications of them are pointed out to him behaviourally or verbally. This often occurs at a time when a patient is being considered for transfer from an institution to a hostel or the community or even for transfer between wards, when some fundamental change of the evaluative system against which his or her behaviour will be measured is about to take place. It is often easy to write off many of the difficulties for which psychotherapy might be appropriate as functions of cognitive inefficiency in the handicapped. Sometimes too these difficulties may be seen partly as functions of physical inefficiency. While it is true that such difficulties can complicate the psychotherapeutic process, they certainly themselves do not preclude it entirely and therapists need to be on their guard lest such elements become rationalisations for discontinuing or not engaging in psychotherapy.

Even by the coarsest criteria, it is apparent that the ordinary population of most institutions may contain significant numbers of patients who have either flagrant mental illness or neurotic difficulties. For example, Craft (1959) estimated that 7% of his sample of 324 patients suffered from mental illnesses and 33% showed personality disorders. O'Connor (1951), using psychometric rather than clinical criteria, judged 12% neurotic and 44% emotionally unstable in a sample of 104 consecutive admissions to a subnormality hospital. Another survey quoted by Gunzburg (1974) surveyed 317 patients in an institution and put 23% of the sample into a category characterised as displaying psychotic features of some kind. Eliminating those who may be most efficiently and humanely treated primarily by physical and pharmacological means, it is the writer's experience that a mean figure of about 20% of patients in the IQ range 40–70 are likely to be helped by psychotherapeutic techniques. This includes some of those just mentioned where physical treatments may be followed up by psychotherapy or counselling.

Over and above this group there is perhaps about another 10% of the population in the average mental deficiency hospital who have periodic exacerbations of emotional difficulty, behavioural upsets or personal crises sufficiently severe to justify psychotherapeutic intervention.

Di Michael & Terwillinger (1953) studied 97 mentally handicapped subjects distributed geographically across the whole of America who had received some counselling or psychotherapy, in order to look at the particular problems of rehabilitation that were dealt with. The age range of the experimental population was from 16 to 65 with the heaviest concentration at the youngest levels from 16 to 21. Median age was 21. There were 53 males and 43 females and in one case sex was unreported. Among these subjects 13 had orthopaedic impairment, 10 had speech defects, 8 had marked personality maladjustment disorders, 4 were cerebral palsied, 4 had defective hearing, 3 cardiovascular conditions and there were 7 with miscellaneous other disabilities. The data outlined below specify the particular problems that were dealt with psychotherapeutically and give a good illustration at a more specific level than is usual, of the applicability of psychotherapy and counselling within the handicapped population, whether or not it is described in more generic terms like 'neurotic', 'psychotic', or 'behaviourally disturbed'. Table 5 illustrates the detailed special problems of these 97 handicapped people.

TABLE 5: Special Problems in Rehabilitation of 97 MR Adults (Di Michael & Terwilliger, 1953)

Personal and interpersonal problems		36
Undesirable personal attitudes	20	
Exaggerated opinions of abilities or wages	7	
Sex problems	5	
Unsustained interest in work	4	
Difficulties in locating suitable jobs		25
Unusual problems in selective placement	12	
Suitable jobs scarce	6	
Illiteracy	6	
Person demanded job with 'sure' advancement	1	
Difficulties due to other disabilities, mostly physical		21
Upsetting family problems		19
Unrealistically high goals for client	8	
Overprotection and indulgence	8	
Serious maladjustment of family	3	
Slowness in learning job		19
Slow manual speed	8	
Slow adaptation to job	8	
Slow adaptation to supervisor	3	
Insufficient vocational training or job experience		7
Previous job failures caused employer resistance		7
Other problems		5
Interim poor health during rehabilitation	4	
Requested job very close to home	1	

Goals of Psychotherapy

It is perhaps useful to start with a rather broad outline of the nature of the operation of giving psychotherapy to the handicapped and of its goals. Slavson (1950) and Beier (1964) have considered that such intervention may take the form of a *cathartic* operation whereby in discussion within group therapy there is 'a discharge of emotions through anger, rage, disgust and quarrelling'. Alternatively, psychotherapy may be used as a *sedative* influence aiming not only at a quieter life for everyone else in the environment, but also at making the clients more capable of dealing calmly with problems in and out of the institution in a socially acceptable way. There is probably a third general type of psychotherapy, the *didactic*, which is aimed explicitly at teaching old dogs new tricks and which is often intermingled procedurally with the sedative type of treatment. Papers by Craft (1965), by Oliver, Simon & Clark (1965) and by Wilcox & Guthrie (1957) illustrate this well. The latter authors describe four features of psychotherapy in which these three main types are intermingled and which seem justifiable on the basis that they extend frustration tolerance and make defectives more socially competent. These are, first, to reduce the suspiciousness felt towards outsiders; second, to release aggression; third, to encourage feelings of self-confidence and initiative in the work situation; and fourth, to develop feelings of responsibility for their actions. Equally clearly it is the case that these are difficult aims to measure as well as to achieve.

Thorne (1948) in an early but wise article, characterised by its own brand of eclecticism, pointed out how much the behaviour of most subnormal persons reflects their own feeling of emotional insecurity in a relatively unstable environment. He pointed out that these patients lack the intellectual resource to compete normally with associates of average intelligence or better and consequently become frustrated and regressive. Many develop undesirable compensatory reactions and they are poorly understood by their normal age peers. His description of what are desirable basic objectives in counselling mental defectives is worth repeating in full:

> (a) accepting the mental defective as being a worthy individual in spite of his defects,
> (b) permitting expression and clarification of emotional reactions,
> (c) patiently teaching him methods for resisting frustration and achieving emotional control,
> (d) outlining standards of acceptable conduct within the ability of each individual,
> (e) building up self-confidence and respect by providing experiences of his success, and
> (f) training the individual to seek help intelligently through counselling when faced with insurmountable problems.

It will be seen that many of these goals make as heavy demands on the therapist as they make on the subject. They also cut across the broad division of cathartic and sedative and didactic treatments. Is it any wonder then that eclecticism of theoretical background must rule the day?

Psychotherapy; Individual or Group?

It is not always useful to adopt the same selection criteria in choosing subnormal subjects for individual therapy as would be relevant in the case of group psychotherapy. To some extent these may be determined in part by the personal style of the psychotherapist and the particular technique of psychotherapy to be used. Factors in the subject which, however, determine individual psychotherapy would be, first, that the subject has marked interpersonal problems which are seen to persist over months and even years and which show signs of continuing to generalise. For example, a patient who has had early experiences in which he has generated hatred of a parent may eventually have had a fight with his supervisor at work, punched up a policeman when drunk or given cheek to bus drivers and so forth and is now taking an anti-authoritarian role within the institution generally or within his extended family. Another kind of difficulty may be exemplified by a patient who may be socially phobic in such a way that she stops going to social clubs in the hospital, then going outside the ward at all, and later has difficulty in eating with others.

A second criterion might be that a subject has too little or no 'release' activities. That is, tension will tend to build up in such a way that the subject cannot displace it on to athletic pursuits, on to personal but socialised rivalries with other patients or people, on to hobbies, or has no alternative ways of releasing emotional tension in a socially acceptable way.

Third, subjects who are suitable for individual psychotherapy do require moderately high arousal levels. They need to be active enough and attentive enough to hear what the therapist is saying, to pick up non-verbal cues such as changes of facial expression, changes of posture, odd bodily movements, intonation and timbre in the voice of the therapist. Argyle's (1967) work makes it clear that non-verbal cues play a very large part in individual communication with such subjects just as they do in the case of normals. Effective communication is not just a function of language and intelligence.

Fourth, it has been found useful to select for individual therapy subnormal subjects who show sufficient emotional variability. Subjects who are overmonotonous in their emotional response and experience not only show too little variability to elicit change in response from those around them, including the psychotherapist, but also may have too limited a range of behaviours to try out new adaptations.

Finally, and perhaps more obviously, subjects who have communication problems in groups clearly need to be treated individually at least in the first instance, often because they are too shy to respond in front of others or because they are deeply inhibited by their stutter, poor articulation or lack of ideas and originality.

There are many occasions when psychotherapy, started with the individual mentally handicapped patient, can be continued in group therapy. Probably the majority of proponents of psychotherapy with the handicapped favour a group approach. The selection criteria for the latter have been reasonably well set out by Slavson (1950) and the writer (Clark, 1977). First, handicapped patients in group psychotherapy must have a minimal capacity for group participation and high 'social hunger'. They must crave to be with others but at the same time be able to demonstrate a balance of aggressive or withdrawn traits. Second, they need to be reasonably responsive to verbal and non-verbal cues given out by the group round them. Third, subjects who clearly require to extend their repertory of social skills probably benefit from the training situation inherent in group activities, where other subjects may act as reinforcing agents of particular behaviours over and above the therapist. Fourth, subjects who are inclined to act out rather than to internalise conflict and difficulty will probably get more scope for therapeutic progress in a group than in the individual situations. It is important too that the *intensity* of a problem in a group can be as much a factor as the *nature* of the problem. Where the problem is very intense in a given individual then this may rule out group treatment and it would be better to deal with this on an individual regime before introducing the subject to the group.

Having looked at the criteria for selection to a group it is easy to move to scrutiny of the advantages of group therapy over individual therapy. The former is clearly economical of time in that one can see several patients simultaneously. It also helps participants develop personal relationships and social ability. Hobbs (1951) has remarked that 'the group situation brings into focus the adequacy of interpersonal relationships and provides an immediate opportunity for discovering new and more satisfying ways of relating to people'. Group approaches tend also to minimise participants' feelings of isolation and insecurity, since being part of a group in which most of the members have fundamentally similar problems can help to give each member of the group feelings of belongingness and acceptance. Also, feelings like embarrassment, anxiety, guilt and the like, which would cause resistance normally tend to be significantly reduced and participants consequently feel more willing to accept and express their inner feelings, thoughts, hopes, disappointments and frustrations. One further advantage of group therapy is that the process of being understood and accepted not only by the psychotherapist but by several people who are honestly sharing feelings and experiences with you tends to be a more potent experience for learning and for finding out the nature of your own personal characteristics than the individual revelations of one-to-one psychotherapy. There is a qualitatively different experience at stake in group psychotherapy, and remarkable inter-patient bonding can occur (often with an increased sense of prestige) in the course of a group's life.

In determining the constitution and size of groups, early writers concentrated on achieving a certain homogeneity either of symptomatology or personality type. With modern developmental/learning approaches this is probably less appropriate than formerly and such a craving for homogeneity in the group may be misconceived. Most authorities consider that 6 to 8 individuals in a group is ideal but therapy can be effective both with smaller groups of 3 or 4 or even with larger groups of 10 to 12. With more individuals than the latter, however, there is a tendency for the group to break into subgroups and Cotzin (1948) found such fragmentation occurring in groups as small as 9, even when the group divided into 7 and 2. The writer's own view is, however, that in cathartic as distinct from sedative or didactic groups, larger numbers give the subjects scope for expression and mutual support and even where fractionation occurs, this can be dynamically important as a statement of the vectors and valencies operating within the group at any given time in relation to a particular topic or anxiety.

There does seem to be some concordance of view that groups should be made up of subjects who, if not homogeneous, are at least balanced in terms of the number of, for example, very aggressive or particularly passive individuals. Slavson (1950) is of the opinion that, in view of the fact that the total group climate is set by the network of feelings among the members and individual relations which form the background for the therapeutic process, selecting the personnel of the group is of the utmost importance. One of the chief aims of grouping in his view is to achieve a permissible quantum of pathology and hostility density. For if these are too high for tolerance by patients who are disturbed as it is, the resultant tensions may be too great not only for the patients but for the therapist as well. Groups need to include therefore people who need to act as neutralisers, who dilute tensions and introduce an element of quiet and control when situations become too difficult or disturbing. Emotions like rage, anger, stress, self-pity, and hopelessness are common and infectious, and unless there is enough rationality and self-control in some of the group members these emotions may become reinforced and over-intensified. Thus the group needs a variety of persons in terms both of syndrome, personality style, arousal level, age and sex.

The writer's experience would suggest that a number of previous authors are correct in suggesting the need for external and rather formal controls determining the course and content of particular group sessions. For example, there is merit in having a definite time limit for each session; for a rule that there should be no display of direct physical aggression towards other members or the therapist; no throwing of objects about the therapy room; some limitation on unnecessarily loud shouting, and no destruction of office equipment. Such behaviours as wandering about the room or even leaving the room from time to time may, however, be useful indices of tension level or dissociation from an internal or situational stress. It is in the determination of rules of this kind that the psychotherapeutic paradigm that the therapist is adopting will make itself clearer. Whatever the paradigm may be, most authors are agreed that the therapist of the mentally handicapped must have a good sense of humour, be able to withstand a certain amount of teasing or personal comment and not to be embarrassed by the participants of the group asking very personal questions. A certain amount of self-disclosure seems almost inevitable and is frequently helpful. It is essential that the therapist be looked upon by the group with respect and as being a sincere, friendly, kind, warm and interesting person. Other rules for the conduct of the group, however, may well be determined by the group and therapist conjointly as treatment proceeds.

Treatment content

It is when he looks in detail at what goes on in treatment sessions with the handicapped that the psychotherapist becomes suddenly aware of his massive eclecticism. This has been especially so since Mundy (1957) endorsed the view of many psychotherapists that the most potent factor in psychotherapy is emotional rather than intellectual comprehension and that the success of psychotherapy depends more on the necessary emotional processes taking place than on their adequate verbalisation. The Truax & Carkhuff (1967) emphasis on 'accurate empathy, non-possessive warmth and genuineness' is well warranted if clients are to enter discussions, respond to and clarify their feelings, set limits to their speech and behaviour, pose questions, accept support, praise and encouragement. Nevertheless, within that context particular techniques and structures may vary enormously. Stacey & De Martino (1957), having reviewed the literature very fully, take the view that there will often be a shift within this context from non-directive or client centred techniques to directive didactic methods. Indeed, most of the recent work looking at the process variables inherent in counselling the mentally handicapped (Stone & Coughlan, 1973; Browning, Campbell & Spence, 1974) has shown such shifts in emphasis and style. The first-named researchers found in later sessions that client and therapist non-problem focussed behaviour and self expression by the therapist increased, and client affective behaviour decreased. The second authors showed how different therapists varied in their approach/avoidance style in relation to clients, particularly dependent on client IQ level, hostility or compliance. Not unnaturally, the clients co-varied in their response styles to the therapist. Unfortunately no work is yet reported on the relationship of therapist success to these process variables. What does seem important, whether in group or individual psychotherapy, is for the therapist to keep a very clear grasp of the specific goals he has set himself for each handicapped patient. Even where the dynamics of the group are themselves inherently interesting this target must never be lost sight of, otherwise the general direction of therapy will become inchoate and random. That must not be mistaken for eclecticism.

There seem to be at least three kinds of eclecticism which operate in the content and structure of psychotherapy with the handicapped. The first of these is an eclecticism about the *setting* in which it takes place. The second is an eclecticism about the *medium used and the techniques* which are predetermined by that medium, and the third is eclecticism of *theoretical standpoint*. So far as the first is concerned, eclecticism of setting, most psychotherapists with the handicapped will be pleased to operate either in the consulting room, the occupational therapy department, the classroom, the ward, the sports field, the art room or the industrial therapy shop. This will be true whether the therapy is individual or group although perhaps it is especially relevant in the case of individual therapy. The setting will be determined as often as not by the fact that it is where the particular patient feels most at ease, is best able to communicate, either verbally or non-verbally, where the behaviours to be modified are demonstrated and where the situation offers that variability of emotional and personal expression that is such an important part of effective therapy. For example, two patients currently in therapy with the writer who are limited to relatively few words in the ordinary way will demonstrate more clearly than otherwise by the aggressiveness of their brush strokes and the violent use of colour and paints how they feel about topics they are being asked about in the art room than elsewhere. In the same way a number of patients who have difficulty with working relationships with their peer group and with supervisors find it hard to abstract and generalise about these in the consulting room but can exemplify by concrete examples in the workshops what sort of situations make them feel uneasy, resentful or aggressive. These situations can then and there be overtly modified by the therapist.

In the same way, the use of art therapy, music therapy, or with children, play therapy, is often especially relevant either as catharsis or sedation. The stimulating or quieting effects of music of a variety of kinds on selected groups of the handicapped is significant especially for those who find it difficult to verbalise their feelings or even to personalise them. Similarly, the use of Makaton and other sign language with non-verbal communicators and the deaf may be much more fitting if it is carried out in the context of a class for sign language in the occupational therapy department than it would be elsewhere in the hospital.

Gesture and non-verbal communication, of course, play a larger part in understanding the attitudes and aspirations of the mentally handicapped than in many other groups. This is especially true with group therapy. For example, one member of a current group whose original behaviour was obtrusively obscene and coprophiliac, in order to test the limits of tolerance of the group, has more recently become affiliated to staff in a new kind of way since he has been given work to do in the physiotherapy department. He is quite unwilling explicitly to align himself with staff since he feels he may lose some loyalties of fellow patients but his behaviour of choosing to sit on successive weeks at group therapy in a chair which progressively gets closer to the therapist is a more obvious behavioural statement of his covert realignment with the staff role. Only recently, the therapist experimentally checked this hypothesis by deliberately removing all chairs from within five feet of his own and the patient, when he entered the room with the others, fetched an upright chair and rather grandiosely set it down immediately adjacent to the therapist such that he was deliberately facing the rest of the group rather than being part of the general semi-circle.

Quite apart from the relative position of members of a group, the individual positioning of and posture within even one chair offer clear statements to the perceptive therapist. One young girl in a recent group, although saying nothing from start to finish of the group which lasted 40 minutes, throughout attended raptly sitting with chin in hands, elbows on table and eyes following every participant in strong contrast with another participant, a male, who while talking fairly freely frequently did so in an offhand, casual and disparaging way with his body half turned away in a chair, legs crossed and picking at his finger ends while looking all the time at some areas outside the enclosing semi-circle of the group.

The eclecticism of technique and methodology is determined in large part by having individual goals for each client whether or not the client is in individual or group therapy. Just as in other aspects of learning, it is important in the psychotherapy of the handicapped to set extremely limited goals which the subject has some possibility of achieving rather than to look for massive acquisitions of more molar aspects of behaviour in the kind of terms one would reserve for normal clients. Examples of the latter might be achieving a better adjustment at home or in work, or coping better with authority figures etc. So far as the mentally handicapped are concerned, an appropriate goal might be instituting a verbal response of one complete sentence to any social approach, reducing social conversation on the part of one patient from a habitual 80 decibel level to nearer 50 or 60 decibels, or training a middle-aged dullard that it is unfair to spend the 50p pieces of other parole patients on herself and leave them with nothing. This is not to say that extension of individual projects of this sort to more generalised levels should not take place. Indeed it is desirable for it to do so within the limits of generalisation posed by the inherent problems of handicap. In group therapy particularly, however, these separate goals often have to be achieved in a context which has its own internal dynamic and where, for example, one may be operating within the terms of a simple operant conditioning reinforcement programme in achieving the goals for one patient in the group. In another, one may be operating very much more within the Kelly system of constructive alternatives in order to improve the self-concept of a patient chronically low in self-esteem by successive positively reinforcing revalidation experiences for that patient. With yet another, one may be concerned to interpret, at least to oneself, the nature of the unconscious factors which are making such demands for realignment with authority figures in the case of Albert quoted earlier. There is therefore an eclecticism of theoretical understanding which runs through every therapeutic episode.

From that point of view, it is not unlikely that at any one time a therapist may be performing in part very much as a Skinnerian operant conditioner, knowing at the same time that in all operant procedures there is necessarily some blurring of the edges at the interfaces of different therapeutic approaches. For example, the reinforcement of individuals leads easily to a scrutiny of the reinforcing patterns within institutions themselves. Baker & Ward (1971) report a study in which a behaviour modification programme was implemented in a living unit within an institution and concluded that 'in the last analysis ... it is not meaningful conceptually to separate the milieu from reinforcement therapy. The availability of reinforcers in the environment, both tangible (as toys or TV) and social (as closer contact with attendants and volunteers) is essential to a total reinforcement therapy program. The reinforcement model becomes helpful in designing the physical milieu so as to provide opportunities and meaningful rewards for learning, along with formal contingencies introduced within that milieu'.

Similarly, it is not unreasonable to adopt models of behaviour in respect of particular patients based on, for example, the Dollard & Miller (1950) notions of learned disordered behaviour and at the same time to accept psychoanalytic notions of conflict at unconscious level emerging as symptomatology. One patient of the writer's, for example, spent a lot of time drawing human figures in therapy, mostly of females, but eventually adding to the figures bunches of flowers or single blooms. These were progressively given more detail until finally there was a violent outburst not of erasing the flowers but of striking them through with bold crayon strokes. The significance of this was only appreciated in psychodynamic terms when it was discovered later that the patient's mother had been an active prostitute and one of his earliest memories was of a client bringing a bunch of flowers to the house. He claimed later to have kicked these about as a child but whether this was a secondary elaboration in terms of his present unconscious aggression towards females and to the 'female' flower symbol of the psychoanalyst could never be clearly established.

Perhaps the most useful theoretical postions for the general guidance of a psychotherapeutic approach in handicap comes from the work of Carl Rogers (1942, 1951) and possibly Harry Stack Sullivan (1953). As a theoretical structure, the work of the former is infinitely more detailed and systematic than that of the latter but at the same time Sullivan's preoccupation with interpersonal relationships and with what he called 'dynamisms' as learned habitual patterns of response (Sullivan, 1953) from which complex habits develop, were important because of their relevance to institutional and community living. The suggestion that these dynamisms are sequential in time and dependent on both a growth process and development of the self, gives them a special relevance to the handicapped because these processes may be independent of chronological age. At the same time, Rogers' proposition that there is a natural course of behaviour development which will result in a healthy, well adjusted person unless it is interfered with by faulty earlier learnings, allows great freedom of route taking to the ultimate developmental goal. The reflexive nature of much of Rogers' therapeutic endeavour bears a strong relationship to Kellyian personal validation or invalidation experience theory. All these therapists ask the respondent or the client to change himself. The therapist has to create conditions in which this will occur. Whereas learning theorists will attempt to explain how the process occurs, Rogers and Sullivan will be more concerned simply to describe it.

It is not unusual in science for one to be able to describe orderly relationships among events and to utilise that knowledge to achieve predictable consequences, even though an adequate explanation of why things work that way may not yet have been developed. The therapist therefore is concerned with sequential events in the therapy of the handicapped and may have to be so over the long term. In carrying out this longitudinal analysis there comes a time when the therapist necessarily will look not only at his own contribution in the group or in the consulting room but will have to take account of the group's dynamic itself, the dynamics of the general environment in the institution and the constant flux of relationships, immediate stresses and underlying subtle enviromental and other influences brought to bear on the patients. These may even be wide-ranging in the form of letters or messages from home and incidental visits from relatives and other third parties.

Where didactic groups may begin with a simple statement such as 'Today we are going to learn how to write letters', followed by a session in which the practicalities of penmanship, the grasp of grammar and the conventions of calligraphy can be literally spelt out, at the same time there will be ample opportunity for subjects to lay bare and explore their attitudes to both the recipients and the senders of letters. The balance of content between the exploration of attitudes and the learning skills in these sessions may swing from week to week.

In cathartic or sedative sessions, however, perhaps one of the easiest ways of opening discussion is for the therapist to introduce a topic through a leading question addressed to one member of the group as a whole. The therapist may then elicit views from all members of the group and throw the matter open to discussion. Occasionally sessions of this sort may be preceded by some boundary setting on the part of the counsellor which might outline one of the areas suggested by the work of Di Michael & Terwilliger (1953) mentioned earlier. Often such sessions allow adequate abreaction and at the same time a good many opportunities for the incidental learning of social subskills which may not be conceived as part of the main operation of the day. It may also subtly reinforce patients' being adequately verbal even if in the process they form small in-groups and factions which lead to more difficulty in interpreting what is going on in the group.

Many sessions of this kind also allow scope for the experiencing of attitudes and emotions which tend to be repressed or denied in day to day life situations. One group therapy incident in recent months in the course of which a lot of sexual and aggressive material was brought up by the group, led to the therapist responding with warm consideration to the complaints of a female patient who maintained that she was always 'put upon' by staff and other patients as the *prima facie* guilty party in various personal and sexual episodes. This undermined the patient's normal front of brash unconcern and sometimes overt aggression to a degree which let her experience for the first time in years 'softer' emotions approaching guilt and remorse. Her experiences in the group which led to a tearful situation in which she was consoled by two other members, who put their arms around her and sat with her, moved her into a new atmosphere of emotional experience which would otherwise have been intolerable, either in her home which was harsh and unrelenting or in hospital where she had set up her own barriers of anger and threat.

Since situations of these kinds can emerge spontaneously and easily in group discussions which range over some of the topics adumbrated, it is easy to see how a more formal role-playing technique can be introduced to such groups. This has value in any of the three categories of therapeutic programme discussed and may take the form of inviting two or more members of the group to act out an employer/employee situation, a father/daughter situation, a mother/son situation or a staff/patient situation focussed on particular areas where there is dispute or disagreement within the group about how events should occur and follow each other. It may be appropriate for the therapist sometimes to assume one of the roles himself or to suggest details of the role to one of the subjects.

Experience has taught that the psychotherapist with patients of limited ability will, however, have to be prepared to vary tension levels within each session and to vary the duration of sessions empirically and within fairly wide limits. There are likely to be days when patients are unprepared to engage in the banter and hurly-burly of dispute and disagreement and when a bland unconcern sits lightly on the group. There will be other days when fisticuffs, tears and laughter blend in the situation which is frequently stressful for the therapist and members of the group but which can result in each learning the other's tolerances and strengths as well as weaknesses. Another episode of recent weeks occurred when the writer was vigorously beleaguered by a female patient who felt that she was being oppressed by the group and the therapist generally, only to find that two or three other members of the group pulled her off and restrained her with unwonted firmness but gentleness. By dint of this she came to recognise how egocentric and socially unrestrained she had become. Happily this awareness generalised until she was able to work again productively in the hospital setting.

Perhaps some of the most difficult crises that face the pyschotherapist with subnormals derive from the fact that patients have limited reality testing opportunities. This is particularly true of their emotional responses within the family and with the opposite sex. Institutional rules, for example, generally prohibit extensive sexual experimentation and visits home tend to be of limited scope and duration. Moreover, they sometimes carry an air of unwonted gentility with the patient being carefully ferried home by a social worker with a modern car and the patient being unusually clean, spruced up and well dressed. Only after several hours when the veneer of sophistication has been sloughed off, a drunken father has wandered in with a half empty chip bag and a slatternly mother is being berated by other members of the family for burning the soup, or for changing the TV programme, does the patient have to cope with the situations where psychotherapy might have made some impact on potential reactions. If there are, however, chances for the patients, whether dealt with originally in groups or individually, to try out new kinds of relationships, a wider range of behaviour or an extended range of emotional responses, then one might expect that some evidence of the beneficial effects of psychotherapy would be forthcoming. It is sometimes fairly easy to see immediate effects, probably of short duration, in patients who are institutionalised. It is discouraging, nevertheless, that when such effects occur they cannot easily generalise to outside situations. In general, exploratory aspects of therapy with the handicapped may well be mediated very much more by 'dynamic' types of theory, whereas the re-learning and re-structuring aspects of pyschotherapy are perhaps best mediated by more deliberate learning theory approaches. It is the latter which will probably take the best account of this longstanding problem of generalisation to the outside, non-institutional setting.

Conclusion

How then is one to rationalise this exercise in therapeutic opportunism, this apparently ill-directed meandering through the garden of theory and practice plucking a bloom here, sowing a seed there, pruning and redistributing with the high-handed assurance of the master gardener? Perhaps, if one changes the metaphor, a representation of the writer's view would be that the psychotherapy of the mentally handicapped is more like building a substantial edifice with bricks of different sizes, hardness and textural characteristics. If they are put together in the correct sequence and so that they fit to make a cohesive pattern, then the structure will stand and may even be extended. One may start to build at different points and all will come right but only if in fact one has an overall plan to guide the activities. This overall plan is the determination of detailed goals for each patient.

In one attempt to present a schematic aetiological model of mental retardation which might guide the process of psychotherapy, Sternlicht (1966) produced that in Table 6. This model seems to the writer, as one schooled in behavioural as well as dynamic psychotherapeutic methods, to be strangely inadequate. In consequence, a third stage, (that below the broken line) is presented by the writer. The so-called bricks comprising the symptomatological syndromes and manifestations chosen by Sternlicht seem far too large for easy

TABLE 6: *A Schematic Etiological Model of Mental Retardation: A Prognostic Index* (after Sternlicht, 1966)

Symptomatological syndrome: manifestations	Etiological influences	Expected outcome of psychotherapy, proportional to etiological influence	Prognostic decision by goals
Intellectual deficit (IQ below 85)	Neurological deficit (Hereditary, prenatal, brain damage)	None	Not indicated
	Cultural deficit (low socioeconomic status, subcultural emphases)	Insignificant	Not indicated
	Emotional disturbances (disturbed childhood, severe environmental stress)	1 Raised IQ (Possible total cure) 2 Resolution of personality maladjustments	Indicated Indicated
Personality maladjustment	Emotional reaction to existing intellectual deficit and concomitant limitations (familial rejection, school failure, job failure, institutional limitations, awareness of inferiority)	1 Personality adjustment 2 IQ unchanged	Indicated Not indicated for this purpose
Behavioural deficit or disorder	Faulty or absent learning of adaptive responses	Establishment or increase in adaptive behaviours Increase in emotional and experienced wellbeing	Specified in some detail

manipulation. The writer, however, suggests a third element in this model which is more easily analysed into its component parts and materials.

With the mentally handicapped one is dealing with 'simple' people in the sense that C J C Earl (1961) used the term. One is inevitably forced therefore to deal at a simple level with simple concepts and behaviours, if necessary simplifying in practical terms as one goes along. It behoves the psychotherapist therefore to begin building his castle with the tiniest bricks available, agreeing that these are the bricks that can be handled both by the therapist and by the client comfortably and easily before putting them together into larger modules. With the exception of some behavioural theories, notably those of Skinner and his colleagues, most theorists in the field of psychotherapy have tended to use too large bricks. Sometimes it seems as if the whole house-sides appear ready made. When, however, one is compelled by experience with mentally handicapped subjects to go back to manipulating the smallest units available and to particularise, it is inevitable that the kind of eclecticism to which attention has been drawn in this chapter is most appropriate. It is this eclecticism which allows these bricks to be put together in a variety of ways and at different rates but nevertheless to form at the end of the day, a substantial edifice with a certain architectural quality, even if the finish is variegated.

The theoretical model presented in Table 7 shows, without being exhaustive, the way in which the therapist has to start with very specific behaviours (Level 1) to be changed, reduced or augmented. With the mentally handicapped, therapy may consist very largely of tackling in an appropriate serial way many behaviours at this basic level. However, if adequate theoretical models are to be formulated and guiding principles, as distinct from behavioural expediencies, are to determine one's progress, then a higher level of conceptualisation becomes appropriate and it becomes easier to adduce a variety of more general theories to determine one's present and future therapeutic behaviour and programme.

Not that it is the therapist's primary purpose to establish principles of behaviour, rather it is to apply established principles to achieve behavioural change. He is, after all, in the business of treating patients rather than theory building. The practising therapist exercising his skills in consulting room, ward or workshop, and drawing his expertise from a miscellany of sources may not necessarily be expected to develop elaborate and carefully organised theories. He simply requires general principles to guide procedure. Ford & Urban (1963) tend to support this general view in their commitment to placing what happens in and results from psychotherapy within the context of general psychology. They, with the writer, counter those psychologists who maintain that psychotherapy represents a special condition sufficiently different from other behavioural situations to require a psychology of its own. In refuting this view, they point out how in general the nature of psychotherapeutic interviews and interactions is such that changes in general behaviour are effected by changes in the patients' response repertoire in therapy.

PSYCHOTHERAPY: AN EXERCISE IN ECLECTICISM 111

TABLE 7: *A Model of Concepts Hierarchically Schematised to allow for Eclectic Intervention in Psychotherapy*

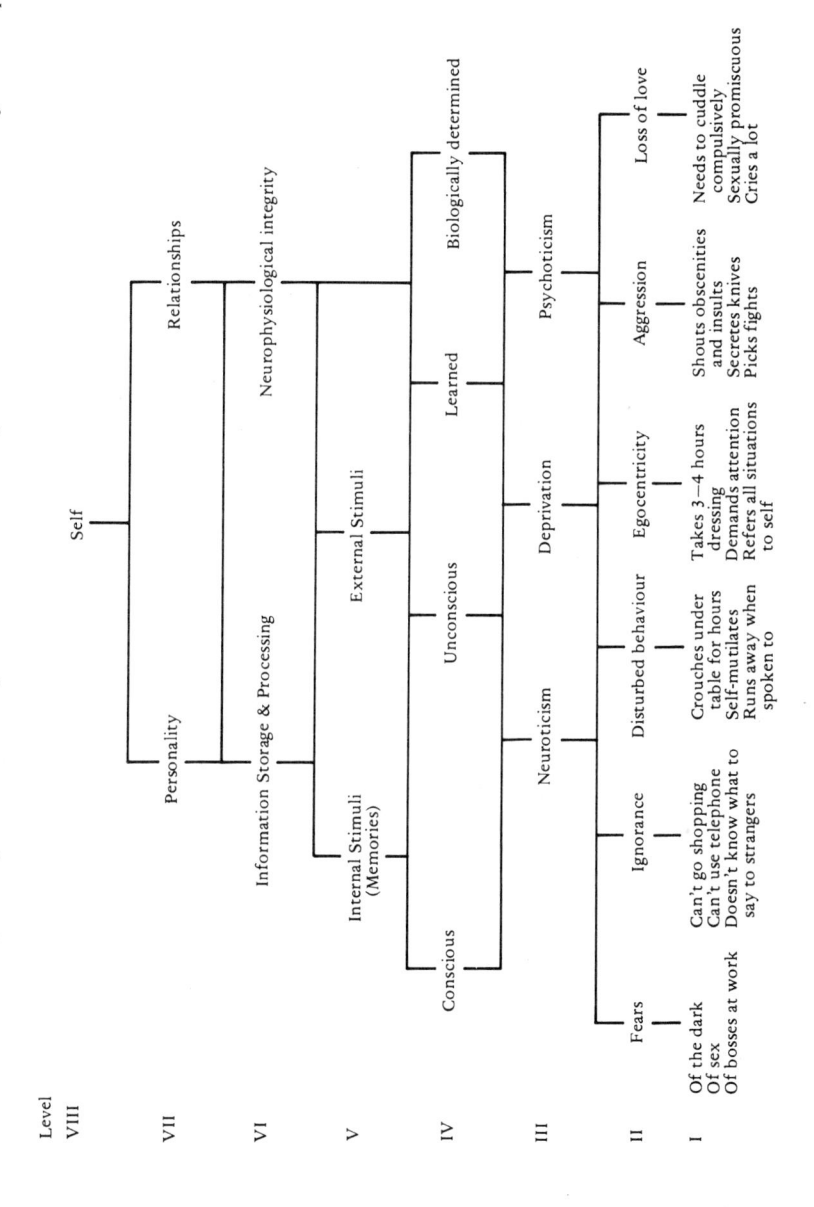

Level		
VIII		Self
VII		Personality — Relationships
VI		Information Storage & Processing — Neurophysiological integrity
V		Internal Stimuli (Memories) — External Stimuli
IV		Conscious — Unconscious — Learned — Biologically determined
III		Neuroticism — Deprivation — Psychoticism
II		Fears — Ignorance — Disturbed behaviour — Egocentricity — Aggression — Loss of love
I		Of the dark / Of sex / Of bosses at work — Can't go shopping / Can't use telephone / Doesn't know what to say to strangers — Crouches under table for hours / Self-mutilates / Runs away when spoken to — Takes 3—4 hours dressing / Demands attention / Refers all situations to self — Shouts obscenities and insults / Secretes knives / Picks fights — Needs to cuddle compulsively / Sexually promiscuous / Cries a lot

This is clearly dependent partly on the therapist's knowledge of the physiological substrate of behaviour which sets the physiological limits of behaviour change. It also involves the question of what behaviour can and cannot be altered, and to what degree, as determined by the limitations of the organism. Similarly, they put the view that the conditions that elicit behaviour must be taken into account when attempting to change the response repertory. Not all behaviours are the result of within-therapy events or of the micro-environment of the treatment room. The sociology and the physical environment of the bulk of the subject's life is an equally important determinant to be taken into account in any theoretical position. As Ford & Urban (1963) say, 'There appear to be three ways in which behaviour can be changed. First, the responding mechanism can be altered. An individual who loses both eyes can no longer see. A patient wrapped in a camisole cannot strike his neighbour. The severing of the vagus nerve reduces in some measure the autonomic reactivity of a person. Second, the situational events that operate to elicit the particular behaviour in the organism likewise can be altered. An angry child can often be distracted by interesting alternatives. Autistic thought sequences in the schizophrenic can often be replaced by interpersonal behaviours if he is confronted by interesting and congenial people. Third, the individual's response repertoire itself may be changed through learning. An American visitor to Japan must alter his driving patterns in order to conform to traffic regulations which differ from those to which he has been accustomed. A patient may come to love rather than fear his father, or the "attitudes" he holds towards himself may be changed'.

Scrupulous eclecticism allows one to analyse the presenting difficulty of the patient in such a way that the appropriate therapeutic steps are taken, using the best theoretical formulation to effect as comprehensive understanding and behavioural change as possible in the circumstances obtaining at the time. That analysis begins by observation at Level I, simple classification at Level II but moves more rapidly toward increasing complexity and inclusiveness of concept at higher levels as the validity of the concepts chosen for understanding is confirmed. Such a principle accommodates the overlap and the differences between the theoretical positions of, for example, Freud, Dollard and Miller, Rogers & Skinner.

Ford & Urban first drew attention to the hierarchical nature of concept organisation related to psychotherapy. Many of the concepts (event classes) that are characteristically employed in personality and therapy theories fall at the higher levels of abstraction (above Level III or IV in Table 7) and therefore stand for or represent large numbers of more specific events. Personality theorists have consequently tended to feel limited in or constrained by the use of small conceptual units, such as Level II, when they have attempted to account for complex interpersonal behaviours. There is, however, no *a priori* reason why one needs to be committed to molar or inclusive concepts in therapy theory all the time. Allport (1937) has proposed that units of all sizes are theoretically legitimate and useful in the conduct of research. It depends on the purpose of the research. No doubt the same could be said of therapy. Allport has suggested groups of units that can be arranged in a hierarchical way, such as 'conditioned response', 'habit', 'attitude', 'trait' and 'personality' with 'self' perhaps being the largest unit of all. Higher order concepts, however, do have the virtue of being more inclusive. It is more convenient and efficient to think about complicated behaviours occurring over a certain amount of time in this inclusive way. For example, one would hardly set out to represent the course of a person's neurotic inability to face large groups by an analysis of the intricate sequences of muscular movements that occurred in his moving from point to point over a series of days. Typically, the more behaviour to which the theorist points the more useful inclusive concepts will be.

There is, however, a significant hazard in conceptualising at these higher levels of abstraction. This stems from the fact that the more removed from relatively discrete observable and confirmable events one becomes, the vaguer and more confused may be the inter-relationships between the concepts at the top end of the hierarchy and the behavioural and situational events at the bottom. The theorist must therefore make explicit the events to which his lower order concepts refer, and if he similarly fails to make clear how higher order concepts are related, at least within his own system, to those of a lower order, confusion will result. The stratifications are relative rather than absolute and may allow some juggling of elements between say, one or two levels. Similarly the model presented does allow the insertion of other elements within levels. Those set out in Table 7 simply describe the nature of the hierarchical model. They are neither inclusive nor definitive. Variations of the elements inserted at different levels may also, of course, vary the interlinking and structural relationships. Table 7 represents only a sample presentation. Many difficulties arise because workers from different schools do not seem to be able to employ the concepts they formulate in a reliable fashion. The same term means different things to different people and these concepts themselves may refer to different events at different times. No wonder communication between therapists can break down.

With models of this kind it is, of course, possible to commit the logical error of reification where the theorist tends to forget that his concepts are abstractions and thinks of them as being real entities. *Events* can really be lost by being 'deep in the unconscious' and *people* can be lost by having 'schizophrenia'. Even Kelly might well have been confused between his real self and his ideal self. Rogers, playing safe, would only have said to him, 'You're not sure who you are?' This must be guarded against.

The great benefit of the kind of eclecticism that has been described in the psychotherapy of the mentally handicapped is that it enables one to enter this kind of schema at the appropriate level without doctrinaire commitment to any particular closed theory of psychotherapy. The need for clinical opportunism, to use a variety of media, the need to effect communication, very often non-verbally with habitually poor communicators, and to start always by dealing with molecular rather than molar behaviour is constantly imposed on the psychotherapist of the mentally handicapped. He must, however, have access to all theories and practices which may make his task more efficient, more humane and more enriching. He has no need to feel guilty about his eclecticism. It ensures that the general principles on which he is operating do not separate him theoretically from the body of work which has been done with non-handicapped patients, and it ensures that these principles do not bind him tightly into the strait-jacket of too doctrinaire a structure which might limit the exercise of his skills or the range of his thinking with this special population. There are, after all, few practitioners of psychotherapy who are not, at least in part, meeting some of their personal needs by the exercise of their skill. And even psychotherapists need some positive reinforcement of their own behaviour. This is especially true for psychotherapists of the mentally handicapped. The eclecticism advocated here should ensure that such reinforcement is regularly delivered.

BIBLIOGRAPHY

Abercrombie, M L J 'Some notes on spacial disability: movement, intelligence quotient and attentiveness', *Develop Med Child Neurol*, 10 (1968) 206

Adler, P T 'Evaluation of the figure drawing technique: reliability, factorial structure, and diagnostic usefulness', *J Consult Clin Psychol*, 35/1 (1970) 52–7

de Ajuriaguerra, J 'Discussion' in S Wapner and H Werner (eds) *The body percept*, (Random House, New York 1965) pp 82–106

Allport, G W *Personality: A Psychological Interpretation*, (Henry Holt & Co, New York 1937)

American Psychological Association 'Ethical standards of psychologists', *Amer Psychol*, (January 1963) 64–71

Ammons, R B et al 'Long term retention of perceptual motor skills', *J Exp Psychol*, 55 (1958) 318–28

Argyle, M *Psychology in Social Problems*, (Methuen, London 1964)

– *The Psychology of Interpersonal Behaviour*, (Penguin, London 1967)

Argyris, C *Personality and Organisation*, (Harper, New York 1957)

Baker, E L and Ward M H 'Reinforcement therapy for behaviour problems in severely retarded children', *Amer J Orthopsychiat*, 41 (1971) 124–35

Ball, T S *Itard, Seguin & Kephart: Sensory Education—a learning interpretation*, (C E Merrill, Columbus Ohio 1971)

Ball T S and Edgar, C L 'The effectiveness of sensory-motor training in promoting generalised body image development', *J Spec Educ*, 1 (1967) 387–95

Barnett, C D, Ellis, N R and Pryer, M W 'Absence of noise effects in the simple operant behaviour of defectives', *Percept Motor Skills*, 10 (1960) 167–70

Barton, R 'The institutional mind and the subnormal mind', *J Ment Subnorm*, 7 (1961) 37–44

Barton, E S 'Operant conditioning of appropriate and inappropriate social speech in the profoundly retarded', *J Ment Def Res*, 17 (1973) 183–91

Baumeister, A A 'The usefulness of the IQ with severely retarded individuals: a reply to MacAndrew and Edgerton', *Amer J Ment Defic*, 69 (1965) 881–2

Beier, D 'Behavioural disturbance', in Stevens, H A and Heber, R F (eds) *Mental Retardation—A review of Research*, (Univ of Chicago Press, Chicago 1964)

Benton, A L 'Right-left discrimination and finger localisation in defective children', *AMA Arch Neurol Psychiat*, 74 (1955a) 583–9

Berkson, G and Landesman–Dwyer, S 'Behavioural research on severe and profound mental retardation', *Amer J Ment Defic*, 81/5 (1977) 428–54

Bricker, D D 'Imitative sign training as a facilitator of word object association with low functioning children', *Amer J Ment Defic*, 76 (1972) 509–16

Bricker, W A 'Identifying and modifying behavioural deficits', *Amer J Ment Defic*, 75 (1970) 16–21

Bricker, W A and Bricker, D D 'Four operant procedures for establishing auditory stimulus control with low functioning children', *Amer J Ment Defic*, 73 (1969) 981–7

Brooks, P H and Baumeister, A A 'Are we making a science of missing the point?', *Amer J Ment Defic*, 81/6 (1977) 543–6

— 'A plea for consideration of ecological validity in the experimental psychology of mental retardation: a guest editorial', *Amer J Ment Defic*, 81/5 (1977) 407–16

Brown, J A C *The Social Psychology of Industry*, (Pelican, London 1954)

Browning, P L, Campbell, D R and Spence, J T 'Counselling process with mentally retarded clients: a behavioural exploration', *Amer J Ment Defic*, 79/3 (1974) 292–6

Brunswick, E 'Representative design and probabilistic theory as a functional psychology', *Psychological Review*, 62 (1955) 193–217

— *Perception and the representative design of psychological experiments*, (Univ of California Press, Barclay 1956)

Burns, R 'Ode to a Louse', 1785

Burt, C *The Backward Child*, (Appleton Century, New York 1937)

Busch, F 'What the Body Says', Scotsman Newspaper, 1972

Caudill, W, Redlick, F C, Gilmore, H R and Brody, E B 'Social structure and interaction process on a psychiatric ward', *Amer J Orthopsychiat*, 22 (1952) 314

Chasey, W C and Wyrick, W 'Effects of a physical developmental prgramme on psychomotor ability of retarded children', *Amer J Ment Defic*, 75/5 (1971) 566–70

Chasey, W C, Swartz, J D and Chasey, C G 'Effect of motor development in body image scores for institutionalised mentally retarded children', *Amer J Ment Defic*, 78/4 (1974) 440–5

Chidester, L and Menninger, K A 'The application of psychoanalytic methods to the study of mental retardation', *Amer J Orthopsychiat*, 6 (1936) 616–25

Clark, D F 'Visual feedback in the social learning of the subnormal', *J Ment Subnorm*, 6/1 (1960) 30–9

— 'A reassessment of the role of the clinical psychologist in the mental deficiency hospital', *J Ment Subnorm*, 14/1 (1968) 3–17

— 'The psychologist and interpersonal relationships in a mental subnormality hospital', *J Ment Subnorm*, 16/1 (1970) 33–44

— 'Body Image and Motor Skill'. PhD thesis, University of Aberdeen, 1975

— 'Psychotherapy with the mentally handicapped'. Unpublished paper, 1977

Clarke, A D B 'Learning and human development', *Brit J Psychiat*, 114 (1968) 1061–77

Clarke, A D B and Clarke, A M *Mental Deficiency: The Changing Outlook*, 3rd ed (Methuen, London 1974)

— 'Prospects for prevention and amelioration of mental retardation: a guest editorial', *Amer J Ment Defic*, 81/6 (1977) 523–33

Clarke, A D B, Clarke, A M and Reiman, S 'Cognitive and social changes in the feebleminded—three further studies', *Brit J Psychol*, 49 (1958) 144–57

Clarke, A D B and Hermelin, B F 'Adult imbeciles—their abilities and

trainability', *Lancet*, 2 (1955) 337—9
Cohen, E A *Human Behaviour in the Concentration Camp*, (Jonathan Cape, London 1954)
Cohen, G *What's Wrong With Hospitals?*, (Penguin, London 1964)
Cohen, H J, Birch, H G and Taft, L T 'Some considerations for evaluating the Doman-Delecato "patterning" method', *Paediatrics*, 45 (1970) 302—14
Connolly, K *Mechanisms of motor skill development*, (Academic Press, London 1970)
— 'Sensory motor coordination: mechanisms and plans', in *Planning for better learning*, ed Wolff and Mackeith, (Heinemann, London 1969)
Cotzin, M 'Group psychotherapy with mentally defective problem boys', *Amer J Ment Defic*, 53 (1948) 268—83
Craft, M *Mental disorder in the defective*. Psychiatric survey among in-patients. *Amer J Ment Defic*, 63 (1959) 829—34
— *Ten Studies into Psychopathic Personality*, (John Wright & Sons, Bristol 1965)
Crossman, E R F W 'Information processes in human skill', *Brit Med Bull*, 20 (1964) 32
Cunningham, R L in Regional Conference on the Hospital Services for the Mentally Handicapped. A Verbatim Report of the Papers given and a Summary of the Discussion. Manchester: Manchester Regional Hospital Board (1971)
Denner, B and Cashdan, S 'Sensory processing and the recognition of forms in nursery school-children', *Brit J Psychol*, 58 (1967) 101
DHSS *Better Services for the Mentally Handicapped*, (HMSO, London 1971)
Di Michael, S G and Terwilliger, W B 'Counsellors' activities in the vocational rehabilitation of the mentally retarded', *J Clin Psychol*, 9 (1953) 99—106
Distefano, M K, Ellis, N and Sloan, W 'Motor proficiency in mental defectives', *Percept Motor Skills*, 8 (1958) 231—4
Dollard, J and Miller, N E *Personality and Psychotherapy: An Analysis in Terms of Learning, Thinking and Culture*, (McGraw-Hill, New York 1950)
Dorry, G W and Zeaman, D 'The use of a fading technique in paired associate teaching of a reading vocabulary with retardates', *Ment Retard*, 11/6 (1973) 3—6
Dubin, R 'Stability of human organisations', in M Haire (ed) *Modern Organisation Theory*, (Wiley, New York 1959)
Earl, C J C *Subnormal Personalities: Their Clinical Investigation and Assessment*, (Bailliere, Tindall & Cox, London 1961)
Edgar, C L, Ball, T S, McIntyre, R B and Shotwell, A M, 'Effects of sensory motor training on adaptive behaviour', *Amer J Ment Defic*, 73 (1969) 713—20
Ellis, N R (ed) *Handbook of Mental Deficiency*, (McGraw-Hill, London 1963)
— 'The stimulus trace and behaviour inadequacy', in N R Ellis (ed) *Handbook of Mental Deficiency*, (McGraw-Hill, New York 1963)
— 'Memory processes in retardates and normals', in Ellis (ed) *Int Rev of Research in Ment Retard*, Vol 4 (Academic Press, New York and London 1970)
— *International Review of Research in Mental Retardation*, Vol 10 (Academic Press, London and New York 1981)
Ellis, N and Sloan, W 'Relationships between intelligence and simple reaction

time in mental defectives', *Percept Motor Skills*, 7 (1957) 65−7

Ellis, N R, Barnett, C D and Pryer, M W 'Operant behaviour in mental defectives: exploratory studies', *J Exp Analysis of Behaviour*, 3 (1960) 63−9

English, H and English, A C A *A Comprehensive Dictionary of Psychological and Psychoanalytic Terms*, (Longmans Green, New York 1958)

Fink, M, Green, M A and Bender, M B 'Perception of simultaneous tactile stimuli by mentally defective subjects', *Journal of Nervous and Mental Disease*, 117 (1953) 43−9

Fisher, S 'Extensions of theory concerning body image and body reactivity', *Psychosomatic Medicine*, 21 (1959) 142−9

Fisher, S and Cleveland, S E *Body Image and Personality*, (Van Nostrand, Princeton 1958)

Fleishman, E A *Structure and Measurement of Physical Fitness*, (Prentice Hall, Englewood Cliffs N J 1964)

Ford, D H and Urban, H B *Systems of Psychotherapy: A Comparative Study*, (John Wiley, New York and London 1963)

Forgays, D G and Forgays, J W 'The nature of the effect of free environmental experience in the rat', *J Comp & Physiol Psychol*, 45 (1952) 322−8

Francis, R J and Rarick, G L 'Motor characteristics of the mentally retarded', *Amer J Ment Defic*, 63 (1959) 292−311

Freedman, S J 'Sensory deprivation: facts in search of a theory', *N Nerv Ment Dis*, 132 (1961) 132, 17

Freeman, R D 'Controversy over "patterning" as a treatment for brain damage in children', *J Amer Med Assoc*, 202 (1967) 385−8

Gardner, W I *Behaviour modification in mental retardation*, (University Press, London 1972)

Gesell, A and Amatruda, C S *Developmental diagnosis*, 2nd ed (Harper & Row, London 1947)

Goffman, E *Asylums*, (Penguin, Harmondsworth 1961)

Goodman, L and Hammill, D 'The effectiveness of the Getman-Kephart activities in developing perceptual-motor and cognitive skills', *Focus on Exceptional Children* 4 (9) (1973) 1−9

Gordon, S, O'Connor, N and Tizard, J 'Some effects of incentives on the performance of imbeciles', *Brit J Psychol*, 45 (1954) 277−87

Grant, G W B, Moores, B and Whelan, E 'Assessing the work needs and work performance of mentally handicapped adults', *Brit J Ment Subnorm*, 19 (1973) 71−9

Gray, D M and Pepitone, A 'Effects of self-esteem on drawings of the human figure', *J Consult Psychol*, 1928 (1964) 453−5

Guetzkow, H and Dill, W R 'Factors in the organisational development of task oriented groups', *Sociometry*, 20 (1957) 175−204

Guetzkow, H and Simon, H A 'The impact of certain communication nets upon organisation and performance in task oriented groups', *Management Science*, 1 (1955) 233−50

Gunderson, E K and Johnson, L C 'Past experience, self-evaluation, and present adjustment', *J Soc Psychol*, 66 (1965) 311−21

Gunzburg, H C 'The role of the psychologist in the mental deficiency hospital',

Gunzburg, H C 'The role of the psychologist in the mental deficiency hospital', *Int J Soc Psy*, 1/4 (1956) 31–6
— *Social Competence in Mental Handicap*, (Baillière, Tindall and Cox, London 1968)
— 'The hospital as a normalising training environment', *J Ment Subnorm*, XVI (1970) 71–83
— *Advances in the Care of the Mentally Handicapped*, (Baillière, Tindall, London 1973)
— *Experiments in the Rehabilitation of the Mentally Handicapped*, (Butterworth, London 1974)
— 'Psychotherapy', in Clarke, A M and Clarke, A D B (eds) *Mental Deficiency: the Changing Outlook*, 3rd edn (Methuen, London 1974)
Haldane, J D 'Child and Family Psychiatry in an Integrated Child Health Service', unpublished SHHD paper, 1972
Halliwell, J W and Solan, H A 'The effects of a supplemental perceptual training program on reading achievement', *Exceptional Children*, 38 (1973) 613–19
Hammer, E F *The Clinical Application of Projective Drawings*, (Thomas, Springfield Ill 1958)
Hammill, D 'Training visual perceptual processes', *Learning Disabil*, 5 (1972) 552–9
Haythorn, W 'The influence of individual members on the characteristics of small groups', *J Abnorm Soc Psychol*, 48 (1953) 276–84
— 'The effects of varying combinations of authoritarian and equalitarian leaders and followers', *J Abnorm Soc Psychol*, 52 (1956) 210–19
Head, H *Aphasia and Kindred Disorders of Speech*, Vol 1 (Cambridge University Press, London 1925)
Aphasia and Kindred Disorders of Speech, (Cambridge University Press, London 1926)
Head, H and Holmes, G 'Sensory disturbances from cerebral lesions', *Brain* 34 (1911) 102–254
Heath, S R 'Railwalking performance as related to mental age and etiological types', *Amer J Psychol*, 55 (1942) 240–7
— 'The relations of railwalking and other motor performances of mental defectives to mental age and etiological types', *Training School Bull*, 50 (1953) 110–27
Hebb, D O *The Organisation of Behaviour: A Neuro-psychological Theory*, (John Wiley, New York 1949)
Heber, R 'Modifications in the manual on terminology and classification in mental retardation', *Amer J Ment Defic*, 65 (1961) 499–500
Heiser, K 'Psychotherapy in a residential school for mentally retarded children', *Training School Bull* 50 (1954) 211–18
Held, R and Hein, A 'Movement produced stimulation in the development of visually guided behaviour', *J Comp Physiol Psychol*, 56 (1963) 872
— — 'Adaptation of disarranged hand eye coordination contingent upon reafferent stimulation', *Percept Motor Skills*, 8 (1958) 87
— — 'Dissociation of the visual placing response into elicited and guided components', *Science*, 158 (1967) 390

Held, R and Schlank, M 'Adaptation to disarranged eye hand coordination in the distance dimension', *Amer J Psychol*, 72 (1959) 603

Held, R and Bauer, J 'Visually guided reaching in infant monkeys after restricted rearing', *Science*, 155 (1967) 718

Hersen, M and Barlow, D H *Single Case Experimental Designs*, (Pergamon, Oxford 1976)

Hill, S, McCullum, A and Sceau, A 'Relation of training in motor activity to development of right left directionality in mentally retarded children', *Percept Motor Skills*, 24 (1967) 363–6

Hobbs, J in Rogers, C *Client-centred Therapy*, (Houghton Mifflin, New York 1951)

Hollis, J H and Carrier, J K 'Research implications for communication deficiencies', *Exceptional Children*, 46 (6) (1975) 405–12

Holman, P 'The relationship between general mental development and manual dexterity', *Brit J Psychol*, 23 (1932) 279–83

Horsley, J S 'The therapeutic climate of staff relationships', *J Ment Subnorm*, 8/1 (1962) 32–45

House, B J 'Problem length and multiple discrimination learning in retarded children', *Amer J Ment Defic*, 78 (1973) 255–61

— 'Scientific explanation and ecological validity: a reply to Brooks & Baumeister', *Amer J Ment Defic*, 81/6 (1977) 534–42

House, B J and Zeaman, D 'Visual discrimination learning in imbeciles', *Amer J Ment Defic*, 63 (1958) 447–52

Hull, C L *Principles of Behaviour*, (Appleton Century Crofts, New York 1943)

Hunter, T D 'Changing patterns of organisation and management', in *New Perspectives in Mental Handicap*, (eds) Forrest, A, Ritson, B and Zealley, A (Churchill Livingstone, Edinburgh and London 1973)

Hymovitch, B 'The effect of experimental variation on problem solving in the rat', *J. Comp Physio Psychol*, 45 (1952) 313–20

Itard, J M G *The Wild Boy of Aveyron*, (Appleton Century Crofts, New York 1932)

Johnson, L 'Body cathexis as a factor in somatic complaints', *J Consult Psych*, 20 (1956) 145–9

Karlsen, S *Executive Behaviour*, (Strombergs, Stockholm 1951)

Katz, D and Kahn, R L *The Social Psychology of Organisations*, (Wiley, New York and London 1966)

Kazdin, A E *Behaviour Modification in Applied Settings*, (Dorsey Press, Illinois 1975)

Kephart, N C *The Slow Learner in the Classroom*, (C E Merrill, Columbus Ohio 1960)

— 'Perceptual motor aspects of learning disabilities', *Exceptional Children*, 31 (1964) 201–6

King, R D, Raynes, N V and Tizard, J *Patterns of Residential Care: Sociological Studies in Institutions for Handicapped Children*, (Routledge and Kegan Paul, London 1971)

Klein, J *The Study of Groups*, (Routledge and Kegan Paul, London 1956)

Kolb, L C 'Disturbances of the body image', in Arieti, S (ed) *American*

Handbook of Psychiatry, Vol 1 (Basic Books, New York 1959) pp 749—69

Koppitz, E M 'Emotional indicators on human figure drawings of shy and aggressive children', *J Clin Psychol*, (October 1966) 466—9

Krasner, L 'Studies of the condition of verbal behaviour', *Psychol Bull*, 55 (1958) 148—70

Lakin, M 'Formal characteristics of human figure drawings by institutionalised and non-institutionalised aged', *J Gerontol*, 15 (1960) 76—8

Landesman-Dwyer, S A 'A description and modification of the behaviour of nonambulatory profoundly mentally retarded children'. Unpublished paper, 1974

Leavitt, H J 'Group communication networks and behaviour of participants', *J Abnorm Soc Psychol*, 46 (1951) 38—50

Le Winn, E B, Doman, G, Delacato, C H, Doman, R, Spitz, E B and Thomas, E W 'Neurological organisation: the basis for learning', in J Hellmuth (ed) *Learning Disorders* Vol 2 (Child Publications Inc, Seattle 1966)

Lewinsohn, P M 'Relationship between height of figure drawings and depression in psychiatric patients', *J Consult Psychol*, 28 (1964) 380—1

Luria, A R *The Role of Speech in the Regulation of Normal and Abnormal Behaviour*, (Pergamon, Oxford 1961)

— *Restoration of Function after Brain Injury*, (Pergamon, New York 1963)

MacAndrew, C and Edgerton, R 'IQ and the social competence of the profoundly retarded', *Amer J Ment Defic*, 69 (1964) 385—90

McCormick, M, Balla, A D and Zigler, E 'Resident-care practices in institutions for retarded persons: a cross-institutional, cross-cultural study', *Amer J Ment Defic*, 80 (1975) 1—17

McFie, J 'Psychological testing in clinical neurology', *J Nerv Ment Dis*, 131 (1960) 383—93

McHugh, A 'Children's figure drawings in neurotic and conduct disturbances', *J Clin Psychol*, 22 (1966) 219—21

Machover, K *Personality Projection in the Drawing of the Human Figure*, (Thomas, Springfield Ill 1949)

Maloney, M P, Ball, T S and Edgar, C L 'Analysis of the generalisability of sensory motor training', *Amer J Ment Defic*, 74/4 (1970) 458—69

Maloney, M P and Payne, L E 'Note on the stability of changes in body image due to sensory motor training', *Amer J Ment Defic* 74/5 (1970) 708

Malpass, L F 'Responses of retarded and normal children to selected clinical measures', Sec I *Perceptual and Response Abilities of Retarded Children*, (S Illinois Univ Press, Carbondale Ill 1959)

— 'Motor skills in mental deficiency', in *Handbook of Mental Deficiency* (ed) Elllis, N R (McGraw-Hill, London 1963)

Mann, R D 'A review of the relationships between personality and performance in small groups', *Psychol Bull*, 56 (1961) 241—70

Maslow, A H *Motivation and Personality*, (Harper Bros, New York 1954)

Matthews, C G 'Quantitative and qualitative differences in retardates and neurologically impaired patients on psychomotor and abstraction ability tasks'. (Paper read at Amer Ass Ment Def Convention, May 1961, Mimeo

Matza, D *Becoming Deviant*, (Wiley & Sons Inc, Univ of California Berkeley 1969)
Merleau-Ponty, M *Phenomenology of Perception*, (Routledge & Kegan Paul, London 1962)
Miles, A E 'Some aspects of culture amongst subnormal hospital patients', *Brit J Med Psychol*, 38 (1965) 171
Minden, H A 'Effect of forced motor activity on learning', *Percept Motor Skills*, 35 (1972) 507–13
Mittler, P (ed) *The Psychological Assessment of Mental and Physical Handicap*, (Methuen, London 1970)
Montessori, M *The Montessori Method*, (Schocken Books, New York 1964)
Morris, P *Put Away: A Sociological Study of Institutions for the Mentally Retarded*, (Routledge & Kegan Paul, London 1969)
— 'Organisational structure and mental subnormality hospitals', *Brit J Ment Subnorm*, 18/1 (1972)
Morrison, D and Pothier, P 'Two different remedial motor training programmes and the development of mentally retarded pre-schoolers', *Amer J Ment Defic*, 77/3 (1972) 251–8
— — 'A remedial sensory motor stimulation programme for pre-school children with developmental deviations', Marin Child Development Centre, California
Mundy, L 'Therapy with physically and mentally handicapped children in a mental deficiency hospital', *J Clin Psychol*, 13 (1957) 3–9
Neman, R 'A reply to Zigler & Seitz', *Amer J Ment Defic*, 79/5 (1975) 493–505
Neman, R, Roos, P, McCann, B M. Menolascino, F J and Heal, L W 'Experimental evaluation of sensorimotor patterning used with mentally retarded children', *Amer J Ment Defic*, 79/4 (1975) 372–84
Nichols, R C and Strumpfer, D J 'A factor analysis of Draw a Person Test scores', *J Consult Psychol*, 26 (1962) 151–61
Nirje, B 'The normalisation principle and its human management implications', in Kugel and Wolfensberger, W *Changing Patterns in Residential Services for the Mentally Retarded*, Washington, Tres Com Ment Retard (1969)
— 'The normalisation principle—implications and comments', *J Ment Subnorm*, 16/2 (1970) 62–70
O'Connor, C 'Effects of selected physical activities upon motor performance, perceptual performance and academic achievement of first graders', *Percept Motor Skills*, 29 (1969) 703–9
O'Connor, N 'Neuroticism and emotional instability in high grade mental defectives', *J Neurosurg Psychiat*, 14 (1951) 226–30
— 'Backwardness and severe subnormality', in Foss, B (ed) *New Horizons in Psychology*, (Penguin Books, Harmondsworth 1966)
O'Connor, N and Tizard, J 'Predicting the occupational adequacy of certified mental defectives', *Occup Psychol*, 25 (1951) 205–11
O'Hara, J 'The role of the nurse in subnormality: a reappraisal', *J Ment Subnorm*, 14/1 (1968) 19–24
Oliver, B, Simon, G B and Clark, B 'Group discussions with adolescent female

patients in a mental subnormality hospital', *J Ment Subnorm*, 11 (1965) 53—7

Osgood, C E *Method and Theory in Experimental Psychology*, (OUP, New York 1953)

Piaget, J *The Origins of Intelligence in Children*, (W W Norton, New York 1952)

Poeck, K and Orgass, B 'The concept of the body schema: a critical review and some experimental results', *Cortex*, 7 (1971) 254—77

Potter, S *One-Upmanship*, (Hart-Davis, London 1952)

Reitman, F *Psychotic Art*, (Routledge & Kegan Paul, London 1950)

Revans, R W 'The analysis of industrial behaviour', in *Automatic Production—Change and Control*, (Inst of Production Engineering, London 1957)

Riesen, A H 'Plasticity of behaviour: psychological series', in Harlow, H F, Wolsey, C N (eds) *Biological and Chemical Bases of Behaviour*, (University of Wisconsin Press, Madison 1958)

Ritchie-Russell, W 'Disturbance of the body image', *Cerebral Palsy Bull*, 4 (1958) 7—9

Roach, E G and Kephart, N C *The Purdue Perceptual Motor Survey*, (C E Merrill, Columbus Ohio 1966)

Rogers, C R *Counselling and Psychotherapy*, (Houghton Mifflin, New York 1942)

— *Client-centered Therapy*, (Houghton Mifflin, Boston 1951)

Ross, R T and Boroskin, A 'Are IQ's below 30 meaningful?', *Ment Retard*, 10/4 (1972) 24

Sarason, S B *Psychological Problems in Mental Deficiency*, 2nd edn (Harper & Row, New York 1953)

Schaefer, H H and Martin, P L *Behavioural Therapy*, (McGraw Hill, New York 1969)

Schilder, P *The Image and Appearance of the Human Body*, (International Universities Press, New York 1950) (Originally published 1935)

Schmitt, R and Erickson, M T 'Early predictors of mental retardation', *Ment Retard*, 11/2 (1973) 27—9

Schneiderman, L 'The estimation of one's own bodily traits', *J Soc Psychol*, 44 (1956) 89—99

SHHD *A Better Life: Report on Services for the Mentally Handicapped in Scotland*, (HMSO, Edinburgh 1979)

Secord, P and Jourard, S M 'The appraisal of body cathexis: body cathexis and the self', *J Consult Psychol*, 17 (1953) 343—7

Sherrington, Sir Charles *Man on his Nature* (Cambridge University Press, 1940)

Shontz, F C *Perceptual and Cognitive Aspects of Body Experience*, (Academic Press, London 1969)

Silverstein, A B and Robinson, H A 'The representation of physique in children's figure drawings', *J Consult Psychol*, 25 (1961) 146—8

Slavson, S R *Analytic Group Psychotherapy with Children, Adolescents and Adults*, (Columbia University Press, New York 1950)

Sloan, W 'The Lincoln-Oseretsky motor development scale', *Genet Psychol Mongr*, 51 (1955) 183—252

Smail, D J 'Values in clinical psychology', *Bull Br Psychol Soc*, 23 (1970) 313—5

Smythies, J R 'The experience and description of the human body', *Brain*, 76 (1953) 132—45

Spitz, H 'The role of input organisation in the learning and memory of mental retardates', in N R Ellis (ed) *International Review of Research in Mental Retardation*, Vol 2 (Academic Press, New York 1966)

Sprott, W J H *Human Groups*, (Penguin, Harmondsworth 1958)

Stacey, C L and De Martino, M F (eds) *Counselling and Psychotherapy with the Mentally Retarded*, (Free Press, Glencoe Ill 1957)

Stanton, A H and Schwartz, M S *The Mental Hospital*, (Basic Books, New York 1954)

Sternlicht, M 'Psychotherapeutic measures with the retarded' in Ellis, N R (ed) *International Review of Research in Mental Retardation*, Vol 2 (Academic Press, New York and London 1966)

Stone, S and Coughlan, P M 'Four process variables in counselling with mentally retarded clients', *Amer J Ment Defic*, 77/4 (1973) 408—14

Strauss, A A and Lehtinen, L E *Psychopathology and Education of the Brain Injured Child*, (Grune & Stratton, New York 1947)

— — *Psychopathology and Education of the Brain-injured Child*, (Grune & Stratton, New York 1951)

Sullivan, H S *The Interpersonal Theory of Psychiatry*, (Norton, New York 1953)

Sutherland, J S, Butler, A J, Gibson, D and Graham, D M 'A sociometric study of institutionalised mental defectives', *Amer J Ment Defic*, 59 (1954) 2

Tansley, A E 'Some aspects of differential diagnosis and treatment in neurologically abnormal children'. Paper read at Conference, January 2, published by the College of Special Education, London, 1968

Thomson, H 'Physical growth' in L. Carmichael (ed) *Manual of Child Psychology*, 2nd edn (Wiley, New York 1954)

Thomson, T and Grabowski, J *Behaviour Modification of the Mentally Retarded*, (University Press, Oxford 1972)

Thorne, F C 'Counselling and psychotherapy with mental defectives', *Amer J Ment Defic*, 52 (1948) 263—71

Tizard, J and Loos, F M 'The learning of a spatial relations test by adult imbeciles', *Amer J Ment Defic*, 59 (1954) 85—90

Tizard, J, O'Connor, N and Crawford, J M 'The abilities of adolescent and adult high grade defectives', *M Ment Sci*, 96 (1950) 889—907

Traub, A C and Orbach, J 'Psychophysical studies of body image. I. The adjustable body distorting mirror', *Archives of General Psychiatry*, 11 (1964) 53—66

Truax, C B and Carkhuff, R R *Towards Effective Counselling and Psychotherapy: Training and Practice*, (Aldine, Chicago 1967)

Wapner, S 'An organismic developmental approach to the study of perceptual and other cognitive operations', in C Scheerer (ed) *Cognition: Theory, Research, Promise*, (Harper & Row, New York 1964a)

— 'Some aspects of a research programme based on an organismic/developmental approach to cognition: experiments and theory', *J Amer Acad Child Psychiat*, 3 (1964b) 193—230

Wapner, S and Werner, H *Perceptual Development*, (Clark University Press, Worcester Mass 1957)

— — 'An experimental approach to body perception from the organismic-developmental point of view', in S Wapner and H Werner (eds) *The Body Percept*, (Random House, New York 1965a) pp 9—25

— — *The Body Percept*, (Random House, New York 1965b)

Webb, R C 'Sensory motor training of the profoundly retarded', *Amer J Ment Defic*, 74/2 (1969) 283—95

Werner, H *The Comparative Psychology of Mental Development*', (Harpers, New York 1940)

Werner, H and Caplan, B *Symbol Formation: An Organismic Development Approach to Language and the Expression of Thought*, (Wiley, New York 1963)

Whelan, E 'Developing word skills: a systematic approach', P Mittler (ed) *Assessment for Learning the Mentally Handicapped*, (Churchill Livingstone, Edinburgh and London 1973)

While, B L, Castle, P and Held, R 'Observations on the development of visually directed reaching', in Hellmuth, J (ed) *Exceptional Infant*, Vol 1 (Bruner/Mazel Books, New York 1964)

White, B L and Held, R 'Sensory and perceptual functions in the cerebral palsied. I. Pressure thresholds and two point discrimination', *J Nerv Ment Dis*, 145 (1967) 53

— — 'Plasticity of sensory motor development in the human infant', *Child Develop*, 35 (1967) 349

Wilcox, G T and Guthrie, G M 'Changes in adjustment of institutionalised female defectives following group psychotherapy', *J Clin Psychol*, 13 (1957) 9—13

Wing, J K 'Institutionalism in mental hospitals', *Brit J Soc Clin Psychol*, 1, (1962) 38—51

Witkin, H A 'Psychological differentiation and forms of pathology', *J Abnorm Psychol*, 70 (1965) 317—36

Witkin, H A, Dyk, R B, Faterson, H F, Goodenough, D R and Karp, S A *Psychological Differentiation*, (Wiley, New York, 1962)

Wittreich, W J and Radcliffe, K B Jr 'The influence of simulated mutilation upon the perception of the human figure', *J Abnorm Soc Psych*, 51 (1955) 493—5

Wolfensberger, W 'Normalising activation for the profoundly and/or multiply handicapped', in Wolfensberger, W, *The Principle of Normalisation in Human Services*, (Leonard Cramford, Toronto 1972)

Yule, W and Carr, J (eds) *Behaviour Modification for the Mentally Handicapped*, (Croom Helm, London and Canberra 1980)

Zaporozhets, A B 'The development of perception in the pre-school child', in Mussen, P (ed) *European Research in Cognitive Development, Monographs of the Society for Research in Child Development*, 30 (1965) 2

— 'Some of the psychological problems of sensory training in early childhood and the pre-school period', in Cole and Multzman (eds) *A Handbook of Contemporary Soviet Psychology*, (Basic Books Inc, New York 1969)

Zarfas, D E 'Moving toward the Normaley Principle in a large government operated facility for the mentally retarded', *J Ment Subnorm*, XVI/1 (1970) 84−92

Zeaman, D 'Experimental psychology of mental retardation: some states of the art'. Invited address to the APA Division 33, New Orleans, August 1974

Zeaman, D, House, B J and Orlando, R 'Use of specific training conditions on visual discrimination learning with imbeciles', *Amer J Ment Defic*, 63 (1958) 453−9

Zigler, E and Balla, D A 'Impact of institutional experience on the behaviour and development of retarded persons', *Amer J Ment Defic*, 82/1 (1977) 1−11

Zigler, E and Seitz, V. 'On "An experimental evaluation of sensori-motor patterning": a critique', *Amer J Ment Defic*, 79/4 (1975) 483−92

Zimbardo, P and Ebbesen, E B *Influencing Attitudes and Changing Behaviour*, (Addison-Wesley, London 1969)